The Ca Family Medicine Handbook

A Quick-Reference Guide for Primary Care Physicians

This page has been left intentionally blank

The Canadian Family Medicine Handbook

A Quick-Reference Guide for Primary Care Physicians

Dr Abdalla Ahmed, MBBS, MRCS, MRCGP, CCFP
Family Physician
WELL Health Medical Centres – Regent
Winnipeg, Manitoba
Canada

Dr Amna Elamin, MBBS, MRCGP, CCFP
Family Physician
WELL Health Medical Centres – Regent
Winnipeg, Manitoba
Canada

2025

Copyright Page

The Canadian Family Medicine Handbook
A Quick-Reference Guide for Primary Care Physicians

Copyright © 2025 by **Dr. Abdalla Ahmed**

All rights reserved. No part of this book may be reproduced, stored in a retrieval system, or transmitted in any form or by any means—electronic, mechanical, photocopying, recording, or otherwise—without the prior written permission of the copyright holder, except in the case of brief quotations embodied in critical articles or reviews.

This book is a work of research and interpretation. While every effort has been made to ensure accuracy, the author and publisher assume no responsibility for errors, inaccuracies, or omissions. The content is provided for educational and informational purposes only and should not be taken as financial, legal, or professional advice. Readers are encouraged to consult qualified advisors for guidance tailored to their specific circumstances.

First Edition, 2025
ISBN: 9798267334884

Published by Dr. Abdalla Ahmed & Dr Amna Elamin
Winnipeg, Canada

Dedication

To our beloved parents,
who have given us everything from the
moment we opened our eyes,
and who continue to give — love, wisdom,
and strength —
without end and without condition.

To our siblings,
our lifelong companions,
who have walked beside us in laughter and in
hardship,
reminding us always that we are never alone.

And to our daughter, Nora,
our future and our light,
the most precious piece of our hearts,
for whom this work is also a legacy of love
and hope.

With deepest gratitude and love,
Abdalla & Amna

Disclaimer

This handbook is intended as a general educational and clinical reference tool for family physicians and other healthcare professionals in Canada. While every effort has been made to ensure accuracy, completeness, and alignment with current Canadian guidelines at the time of publication, medicine is a rapidly evolving field. Recommendations, drug dosages, and clinical practices may change as new evidence emerges.

The authors and publishers make no representations or warranties about the accuracy, reliability, or completeness of the content, and accept no responsibility or liability for any errors, omissions, or outcomes resulting from the use of this material.

This handbook is not a substitute for professional medical judgment. Physicians are expected to use their own clinical judgment in each individual case, considering the unique circumstances of their patients. Where appropriate, clinicians should consult up-to-date guidelines, product monographs, and specialist colleagues before making management decisions.

Medication names, doses, and regimens provided in this handbook are for reference purposes only and should be verified against current formularies and product information. Patients should never rely on this book as a source of medical advice; they should consult their own physician or qualified healthcare provider for diagnosis and treatment of medical conditions.

Use of this handbook signifies understanding and acceptance of these terms.

CONTENTS

Preface 13

Part I – Foundations of Family Medicine . 15

1. Introduction to Canadian Family Medicine 16
2. Clinical Approach in Family Medicine 20
3. Preventive Care & Screening 23

Part II – Symptom-Based Approach 27

4. Chest Pain 29
5. Shortness of Breath 35
6. Cough & Hemoptysis 40
7. Abdominal Pain (Acute & Chronic) 45
8. Headache (acute and chronic) 50
9. Back Pain 55
10. Fatigue 61
11. Dizziness & Vertigo 66
12. Rash & Skin Lesions 71
13. Fever of Unknown Origin 77
14. Depression, Anxiety & Insomnia 83
15. Pediatric Presentations 89
16. Geriatric Presentations 95

Part III – Clinical Systems 101

Section 1: Cardiovascular Medicine 103

17. Hypertension 104

18. Dyslipidemia & ASCVD Prevention 107

19. Angina & Acute Coronary Syndrome (ACS) 110

20. Heart Failure (HFrEF & HFpEF) 113

21. Arrhythmias (AF, SVT, Bradyarrhythmias) 118

22. Stroke & Transient Ischemic Attack (TIA) 122

Section 2: Respiratory Medicine 127

23. Asthma 128

24. Chronic Obstructive Pulmonary Disease (COPD) 132

25. Pneumonia 136

26. Tuberculosis (TB) 140

27. Pulmonary Embolism (PE) 144

28. Obstructive Sleep Apnea (OSA) 148

Section 3: Endocrinology & Metabolism 153

29. Diabetes Mellitus 154

30. Thyroid Disease 158

31. Adrenal & Pituitary Disorders 161

32. Osteoporosis & Bone Health 165

33. Obesity Management 169

34. Vitamin D Deficiency 173

Section 4: Gastroenterology 177

35. GERD, Dyspepsia & Peptic Ulcer Disease (PUD) 178

36. Irritable Bowel Syndrome (IBS) vs Inflammatory Bowel Disease (IBD) 182

37. Constipation & Diarrhea 186

38. Celiac Disease 190

39. Hepatitis B & C 194

40. Non-Alcoholic Fatty Liver Disease (NAFLD) 198

Section 5: Renal & Urology 203

41. Chronic Kidney Disease (CKD) 204

42. Hematuria & Proteinuria 208

43. Benign Prostatic Hyperplasia (BPH) & Prostatitis 212

44. Urinary Tract Infections (UTIs): Pediatric, Male, Female & Recurrent 216

45. Nephrolithiasis (Kidney Stones) 220

Section 6: Women's Health 225

46. Contraception Overview 226

47. Menstrual Disorders (Dysmenorrhea, Abnormal Bleeding, Amenorrhea) 230

48. Antenatal & Postnatal Care in Family Practice 235

49. Menopause & Hormone Replacement Therapy (HRT).. 239

50. Breast Disorders (Mastitis, Fibroadenoma, Cancer Screening).. 243

Section 7: Men's Health 247

51. Prostate Health (BPH, Cancer Screening) 248

52. Erectile Dysfunction (ED) 252

53. Hypogonadism 256

Section 8: Pediatrics 261

54. Well Child Care & Immunizations 262

55. Common Pediatric Infections 269

56. Pediatric Respiratory Conditions 276

57. Pediatric GI & Nutrition 283

58. Pediatric Dermatology 290

59. Pediatric Neurology 298

60. Pediatric Musculoskeletal & Injuries 305

61. Pediatric Mental Health 311

62. Adolescent Medicine 318

Section 9: Geriatric Medicine 325

63. Dementia, Delirium, Depression in the Elderly 326

64. Frailty & Falls Assessment 331

65. Polypharmacy Management 335

66. Palliative and End-of-Life Care 339

Section 11: Dermatology 343

72. Eczema, Psoriasis, Urticaria 344

73. Skin Infections (Bacterial, Fungal, Viral) 349

74. Skin Cancers (BCC, SCC, Melanoma) 354

75. Acne & Rosacea 358

76. Alopecia 362

Section 12: Mental Health & Psychiatry. 367

77. Depression 368

78. Anxiety & Panic Disorders 372

79. Bipolar Disorder 376

80. Psychosis & Schizophrenia 380

81. Suicide Risk Assessment 384

Section 13: Infectious Diseases 389

82. Common Community Infections 390

83. STI Screening & Management 396

84. HIV, Hepatitis B & C 401

85. Travel Medicine Essentials 407

This page has been left intentionally blank

Preface

Family medicine is the cornerstone of Canada's healthcare system. As family physicians, we care for patients at every stage of life, across all care settings, and for a vast range of health concerns. This unique scope makes family medicine both deeply rewarding and intellectually challenging, requiring both breadth and adaptability.

This handbook was created as a **concise, practical resource for Canadian family doctors**. It is not a replacement for comprehensive textbooks or specialist guidelines, but a **quick-reference guide** designed to support physicians in day-to-day clinical decision-making at the point of care.

The book is organized to mirror real-world practice:

- **Foundations of family medicine** review our role, communication strategies, and preventive care.
- **Symptom-based** s guide initial assessment, red flags, and practical office management.
- **System-based disease sections** summarize key conditions across major specialties, with emphasis on what to do in the office, when to refer to

emergency care, and when specialist involvement is required.
- **Dedicated sections on mental health, pediatrics, geriatrics, dermatology, and infectious diseases** address some of the most common and high-impact presentations in Canadian primary care.

Where possible, recommendations are based on **Canadian guidelines** such as the CTFPHC, Hypertension Canada, CDA, CPS, CTS, and IDSA (Canadian adaptations). Each blends **narrative summaries** with **bullet-point checklists**, so readers can quickly find essential information.

This handbook was written for the **busy family physician** — whether in clinic, hospital, emergency, or rural/remote settings. It is equally relevant for residents learning the discipline, early-career physicians establishing their practice, and seasoned practitioners looking for a reliable pocket companion.

We dedicate this book to our patients, who entrust us with their care and remind us daily of the privilege it is to serve as their family doctors.

Dr. Abdalla Ahmed
Dr. Amna Elamin
Winnipeg, Manitoba

Part I – Foundations of Family Medicine

1. Introduction to Canadian Family Medicine

Family medicine is the backbone of the Canadian healthcare system. It provides comprehensive, continuous, and coordinated care across the lifespan, addressing health needs from infancy to end of life. Unlike specialty care, family medicine emphasizes the whole person, family, and community context.

The Role of the Family Physician

Family physicians serve as the first point of contact for patients, offering both acute and chronic care. They function as:

- **Primary caregivers**: managing common illnesses and preventive health.
- **Coordinators**: guiding patients through referrals, investigations, and specialist care.
- **Continuity providers**: building long-term therapeutic relationships.
- **Comprehensive clinicians**: addressing physical, mental, and social health.

Scope of Practice Across Provinces

The scope of practice in family medicine is broad but varies across provinces and communities:

- **Office-based care**: preventive medicine, chronic disease management, minor procedures.
- **Hospital care**: inpatient medicine, obstetrics, emergency shifts (in many rural/remote settings).
- **Community services**: palliative care, home visits, nursing home care.
- **Procedural work**: suturing, joint injections, skin lesion removal; in rural areas, may include C-sections and anesthesia.
- **Variation**: Scope depends on physician training, local needs, and provincial policies.

Organization of the Canadian Healthcare System

Canada's healthcare operates under the **Canada Health Act**, ensuring universal coverage for medically necessary services.

- **Publicly funded, single-payer system (Medicare).**

- Delivered and managed by **provinces/territories**, with federal funding and oversight.
- **Access**: Patients need a valid provincial health card.
- **Coverage**: Physician services and hospital care are publicly funded; medications, dental, vision, and allied health usually require private or employer insurance.
- **Primary care entry point**: Most patients access care first through their family doctor, who acts as a **gatekeeper** to specialist services.

Indigenous Health, Equity, and Cultural Safety

Family physicians in Canada must be mindful of health disparities and the importance of culturally safe care.

- **Indigenous health**: Indigenous communities face disproportionate burdens of chronic disease, mental health challenges, and access barriers. Historical trauma and systemic inequities contribute to ongoing health gaps.
- **Equity in practice**: Family doctors need to account for social determinants

of health — income, housing, education, food security.
- **Cultural safety**: Goes beyond cultural competence; requires ongoing self-reflection, recognizing systemic power imbalances, and providing care that patients perceive as safe and respectful.
- **Newcomers and refugees**: Often present with unique health needs (immunizations, trauma, language barriers, settlement challenges).

2. Clinical Approach in Family Medicine

Family medicine consultations are unique. They balance time efficiency with the need to understand the patient's broader context. Unlike specialty care, family physicians often see patients over many years, which builds trust and continuity but also requires skill in managing uncertainty and wide-ranging problems.

The Patient-Centred Clinical Method

This Canadian model emphasizes the patient's experience and context alongside the disease.

- Explore illness experience: patient's ideas, concerns, expectations.
- Understand patient's context: family, work, culture, social supports.
- Find common ground: negotiate shared goals and management plans.
- Strengthen relationship: continuity builds trust and adherence.

Consultation Models

Different frameworks help structure encounters.

- **SOAP (Subjective, Objective, Assessment, Plan):** widely used for documentation.
- **Calgary–Cambridge Guide:** structured approach to consultation skills.
- **ICE (Ideas, Concerns, Expectations):** simple model to explore patient perspective.
- **BATHE (Background, Affect, Trouble, Handling, Empathy):** especially useful in psychosocial consultations.

Communication Skills

Good communication is at the heart of family medicine.

- **Active listening** and empathy are key.
- Use **plain language**; avoid jargon.
- **Motivational interviewing**: collaborative style for behaviour change (smoking cessation, lifestyle).
- **Breaking bad news (SPIKES):**
    - Setting → Privacy, time, support.
    - Perception → Explore patient's understanding.

- Invitation → Ask how much they want to know.
- Knowledge → Give clear information.
- Empathy → Respond to emotions.
- Strategy → Plan next steps together.

Documentation, Medico-Legal Issues, and Consent

Accurate and thorough documentation protects both patient and physician.

- Document history, examination, differential, plan, and patient's response.
- Record discussions of risks, benefits, and alternatives when obtaining consent.
- Note patient refusals and the advice given.
- Align with **provincial College standards** and medico-legal frameworks.
- **Informed consent** must include capacity, voluntariness, and adequate information.

3. Preventive Care & Screening

Preventive care is a defining feature of family medicine in Canada. Family physicians are often the first to discuss screening and prevention, using national guidelines such as those from the **Canadian Task Force on Preventive Health Care (CTFPHC)** and the **National Advisory Committee on Immunization (NACI)**. The emphasis is on **evidence-based interventions** that provide real benefit, while avoiding unnecessary or harmful tests.

CTFPHC Guidelines Overview

The Canadian approach prioritizes **shared decision-making** and screening only when evidence supports improved outcomes.

- Focus on reducing morbidity and mortality, not just detecting disease.
- Avoid overdiagnosis and overtreatment.
- Engage patients in choosing whether to screen, especially when benefits are modest.

Immunizations

Immunizations are among the most effective preventive interventions. Schedules vary slightly by province, but are guided nationally by NACI.

- **Children:** DTaP, IPV, Hib, MMR, varicella, meningococcal, pneumococcal, HPV.
- **Adults:**
    - Tdap booster every 10 years.
    - Annual influenza vaccine.
    - Shingles vaccine (Shingrix) for adults >50 years.
    - Pneumococcal vaccines (PCV20 or PPSV23) for adults >65 or at risk.
- **Special populations:** Travel vaccines (yellow fever, typhoid, hepatitis A/B) and occupational vaccines (healthcare, lab workers).

Cancer Screening

Cancer screening recommendations are tailored to age and risk factors.

- **Breast cancer:** Mammogram every 2–3 years for women aged 50–74.

- **Cervical cancer:** Pap test every 3 years from age 25–69 (many provinces now moving to HPV testing).
- **Colorectal cancer:** FIT test every 2 years for adults aged 50–74.
- **Lung cancer:** Low-dose CT for high-risk adults aged 55–74 with ≥30 pack-year smoking history, current or quit within 15 years.
- **Prostate cancer:** Routine PSA screening not recommended; offer only through shared decision-making if requested.

Cardiovascular Risk Screening

Cardiovascular disease remains the leading cause of death in Canada. Screening focuses on risk assessment rather than single numbers.

- **Blood pressure:** Screen all adults ≥18 years, frequency based on risk (every 1–5 years).
- **Lipids:** Screen men ≥40, women ≥50 or post-menopausal, and earlier if high risk.
- **Diabetes:** Screen with HbA1c every 3–5 years in adults ≥40, earlier if risk factors (obesity, high-risk ethnic groups, family history, GDM).
- **Obesity:** BMI and waist circumference at routine visits.

Osteoporosis & Fracture Risk

Fractures are a major source of morbidity in older adults.

- **Screen women ≥65 years** with DXA scan.
- **Men ≥70 years** may also benefit, though evidence is less strong.
- Use **FRAX** tool to estimate fracture risk in patients with risk factors.

Mental Health & Substance Use Screening

Mental health and addictions are common but often underdiagnosed in primary care.

- **Depression/anxiety:** Screen at-risk groups using tools such as PHQ-9 and GAD-7.
- **Alcohol misuse:** Use AUDIT-C or CAGE.
- **Tobacco:** Ask at every visit; use Ask–Advise–Act framework.
- **Other substances:** Screen when risk is suspected, especially opioids and cannabis.

Part II – Symptom-Based Approach

This page has been left intentionally blank

4. Chest Pain

Introduction

Chest pain is one of the most challenging and high-stakes presentations in family practice. While many cases are benign (musculoskeletal, reflux, anxiety), some represent life-threatening emergencies (acute coronary syndrome, pulmonary embolism, aortic dissection). The family physician's role is to rapidly identify red flags, stabilize the patient if needed, and determine whether the case can be safely managed in the office or requires urgent hospital referral.

Differential Diagnosis

Cardiac

- Acute coronary syndrome (MI, unstable angina)
- Stable angina
- Pericarditis
- Aortic dissection

Respiratory

- Pulmonary embolism
- Pneumothorax (spontaneous, tension)

- Pneumonia, pleuritis

Gastrointestinal

- GERD, esophagitis
- Peptic ulcer disease
- Gallbladder disease (biliary colic, cholecystitis)

Musculoskeletal

- Costochondritis
- Muscle strain
- Rib fracture

Psychiatric/Other

- Panic attack, anxiety
- Herpes zoster (pre-eruption)

What to Do in the Office

1. Rapid Initial Assessment

- Check **ABCs** (airway, breathing, circulation).
- Measure **vitals**: BP (both arms if possible), HR, RR, SpO$_2$, temperature.
- Observe: pallor, diaphoresis, distress level.

2. Focused History

- Onset, character, location, radiation, duration.
- Associated symptoms: SOB, syncope, diaphoresis, nausea.
- Risk factors: HTN, diabetes, smoking, dyslipidemia, family history, prior CAD.

3. Focused Exam

- Cardiovascular: heart sounds, murmurs, JVP, pulses.
- Respiratory: breath sounds, wheeze, crackles, asymmetry.
- Chest wall palpation (reproducible pain = more likely MSK).
- GI: epigastric tenderness, RUQ tenderness.

4. In-Office Investigations (if available)

- **ECG:** Do on all patients with suspected ACS or cardiac chest pain.
- **Pulse oximetry:** Assess oxygen saturation.
- **POC glucose** (rule out diabetic complication if symptomatic).
- **POC troponin:** If available in clinic (not universal).

5. Initial Management (office level)

- **If ACS suspected: Give ASA 160–325 mg chewable immediately**.

- **Sublingual nitroglycerin** if SBP >90 mmHg and no RV infarct suspected.
- Oxygen only if SpO$_2$ <90%.
- Arrange **EMS transfer to ED immediately**.

When to Refer to ED (Call EMS, do not send by car)

- Any red flags or unstable vitals.
- Suspected: ACS, pulmonary embolism, aortic dissection, tension pneumothorax, esophageal rupture.
- Severe or worsening chest pain with abnormal ECG or troponin (if available).

When to Refer to Specialists (Non-Urgent)

- **Cardiology:**
  - Stable angina requiring risk stratification or further work-up.
  - Abnormal ECG findings (e.g., Q waves, LVH, arrhythmias).
  - Heart failure or structural heart disease with chest pain.
- **Gastroenterology:**

- Refractory GERD/dyspepsia not responding to PPI.
- **Psychiatry/CBT referral:**
  - Panic attacks, anxiety disorder causing recurrent chest pain once organic causes excluded.

When to Manage in Primary Care

- **Musculoskeletal chest pain** (costochondritis, strain) → NSAIDs, reassurance, physiotherapy if recurrent.
- **GERD-related pain** → PPI trial, lifestyle advice.
- **Anxiety/panic** → breathing techniques, short-term anxiolytic if indicated, CBT referral.
- **Herpes zoster (pre-eruptive pain with rash appearing later)** → antivirals if within 72h.

Pocket Box – Office Chest Pain Quick Reference

- **Step 1:** Vitals, ABCs, rapid history.
- **Step 2:** ECG + SpO_2 (if available).
- **Step 3:**

- o **Unstable/red flag:** ASA → nitro (if safe) → EMS transfer.
- o **Stable, benign features:** Manage cause (MSK, GERD, anxiety).
- **Step 4:** Arrange referral (cardiology, GI, psychiatry) if indicated.

5. Shortness of Breath

Introduction

Shortness of breath (dyspnea) is a frequent presentation in family medicine. It may arise from cardiac, respiratory, metabolic, or even psychological causes. In the office, the physician must rapidly identify patients in distress who require urgent hospital transfer, while also managing stable cases safely in primary care.

Differential Diagnosis

Respiratory

- Asthma, COPD exacerbation
- Pneumonia, bronchitis
- Pulmonary embolism
- Interstitial lung disease
- Pneumothorax

Cardiac

- Heart failure (acute or chronic)
- Ischemic heart disease (MI, unstable angina)
- Arrhythmias
- Pericardial effusion/tamponade

Other Causes

- Anemia
- Obesity, deconditioning
- Anxiety/panic disorder
- Metabolic acidosis (DKA, sepsis)

What to Do in the Office

1. Rapid Initial Assessment

- Check **ABCs** immediately.
- Vitals: HR, BP, RR, O_2 sat, temperature.
- Look for: use of accessory muscles, cyanosis, inability to speak full sentences.

2. Focused History

- Onset: acute vs chronic.
- Associated symptoms: cough, wheeze, chest pain, fever, orthopnea, leg swelling.
- Past history: asthma, COPD, cardiac disease, clotting risk factors.

3. Focused Exam

- Respiratory: wheeze, crackles, decreased breath sounds, asymmetry.

- Cardiac: JVP, murmurs, gallops, peripheral edema.
- General: pallor (anemia), agitation, cachexia.

4. In-Office Investigations (if available)

- Pulse oximetry.
- ECG: for suspected cardiac cause.
- Peak flow or spirometry (if asthma/COPD, when stable).
- Chest X-ray, bloodwork → usually arranged urgently through hospital, not office.

5. Initial Management (office level)

- Oxygen if SpO_2 <90%.
- Bronchodilator therapy for suspected asthma/COPD exacerbation (salbutamol ± ipratropium).
- Oral prednisone for moderate–severe asthma/COPD flare.
- Antibiotics if pneumonia strongly suspected and patient stable for outpatient treatment.

When to Refer to ED (Call EMS)

- Severe respiratory distress (inability to speak, altered LOC, exhaustion).
- SpO_2 <90% despite oxygen.

- Suspected pulmonary embolism, pneumothorax, acute heart failure, ACS.
- Rapidly worsening symptoms, unstable vitals.

When to Refer to Specialists (Non-Urgent)

- **Respirology:** recurrent or severe asthma, uncontrolled COPD, interstitial lung disease.
- **Cardiology:** heart failure, suspected ischemia, unexplained dyspnea with abnormal ECG/echo.
- **Hematology/Internal Medicine:** unexplained anemia causing dyspnea.

When to Manage in Primary Care

- Mild asthma or COPD exacerbation responding to inhaled therapy.
- Community-acquired pneumonia in a stable patient (no hypoxia, can tolerate oral intake, no comorbidities requiring admission).
- Anxiety-related dyspnea once organic causes are ruled out.

- Chronic conditions with stable symptoms (e.g., mild COPD, anemia under treatment).

Pocket Box – Office Dyspnea Quick Reference

- **Step 1:** ABCs, vitals, SpO_2.

- **Step 2:** Rapid history + focused exam (respiratory + cardiac).

- **Step 3:**

    - **Unstable/red flag:** Oxygen → bronchodilators if asthma/COPD → EMS transfer.

    - **Stable:** Treat cause (pneumonia antibiotics, mild asthma/COPD therapy, anxiety reassurance).

- **Step 4:** Refer specialist (respirology, cardiology) if needed.

6. Cough & Hemoptysis

Introduction

Cough is one of the most common reasons for visits in family practice. It may be acute, subacute, or chronic, and ranges from benign viral infections to serious conditions like pneumonia or lung cancer. Hemoptysis (coughing blood) is less common but always requires careful assessment. The family physician must distinguish between cases that can be managed in the office and those needing urgent referral.

Differential Diagnosis

Cough

- **Acute (<3 weeks):** viral URTI, acute bronchitis, pneumonia, asthma/COPD exacerbation.
- **Subacute (3–8 weeks):** post-infectious cough, pertussis, asthma.
- **Chronic (>8 weeks):** asthma, COPD, GERD, post-nasal drip, ACE inhibitor side effect, lung cancer, interstitial lung disease.

Hemoptysis

- Infection: bronchitis, pneumonia, TB.
- Chronic lung disease: COPD, bronchiectasis.
- Malignancy: lung cancer.
- Pulmonary embolism.
- Rare: vasculitis, mitral stenosis.

What to Do in the Office

1. Rapid Initial Assessment

- Vitals: HR, BP, RR, O_2 sat, temperature.
- Is the patient hypoxic, tachypneic, unstable?
- Estimate severity of hemoptysis (streaks vs cupful).

2. Focused History

- Duration of cough: acute, subacute, chronic.
- Character: dry vs productive; blood present?
- Associated symptoms: fever, chest pain, weight loss, night sweats.
- Smoking history, TB exposure, occupational exposures.
- Medication history (ACE inhibitors).

3. Focused Exam

- Respiratory: wheeze, crackles, bronchial breathing, decreased sounds.
- Cardiac: murmurs, JVP (pulmonary hypertension/CHF).
- ENT: post-nasal drip, sinus tenderness.

4. In-Office Investigations (if available)

- Pulse oximetry.
- Chest X-ray (if accessible same-day).
- Sputum sample if infection suspected.
- Consider CBC (infection, anemia).

5. Initial Management

- **Acute viral cough/bronchitis:** reassurance, fluids, symptomatic treatment.
- **Asthma/COPD:** bronchodilators, steroids if exacerbation.
- **Pneumonia (stable):** antibiotics in office, close follow-up.
- **ACE inhibitor cough:** switch drug.

When to Refer to ED (Urgent)

- Massive hemoptysis (>200 mL in 24 hrs or rapid ongoing bleed).
- Respiratory distress, hypoxia (SpO$_2$ <90%).
- Suspected pulmonary embolism with hemodynamic instability.

- Severe pneumonia/sepsis.

When to Refer to Specialists (Non-Urgent)

- **Respirology:** chronic cough unexplained by initial work-up, suspected interstitial lung disease, bronchiectasis, or moderate hemoptysis.
- **Oncology/Respirology:** abnormal chest imaging suspicious for lung cancer.
- **ENT:** chronic post-nasal drip not responsive to therapy.
- **Cardiology:** hemoptysis due to valvular heart disease (rare).

When to Manage in Primary Care

- Viral URTI/post-viral cough.
- Mild asthma or COPD flare responding to office treatment.
- Stable, mild pneumonia (normal oxygen, no sepsis, able to tolerate oral intake).
- ACE inhibitor–related cough.
- Anxiety-related "habit cough."

Pocket Box – Office Cough & Hemoptysis Quick Reference

- **Step 1:** Vitals, ABCs, estimate severity of hemoptysis.
- **Step 2:** History (duration, sputum, risk factors), focused exam.
- **Step 3:**
  - **Unstable/red flag:** hypoxia, massive hemoptysis, sepsis → EMS transfer.
  - **Stable:** CXR if available, treat cause (antibiotics, bronchodilators, supportive).
- **Step 4:** Specialist referral for chronic unexplained cough, abnormal imaging, or moderate hemoptysis.

7. Abdominal Pain (Acute & Chronic)

Introduction

Abdominal pain is a very common presentation in family medicine. Most cases are benign, but a small proportion represent surgical emergencies. The family physician's role in the office is to identify red flags, provide initial stabilization when required, and distinguish between conditions that can be managed in primary care versus those needing urgent hospital or specialist evaluation.

Differential Diagnosis

Acute Causes

- Appendicitis
- Cholecystitis, biliary colic
- Bowel obstruction, perforation
- Diverticulitis
- Pancreatitis
- Gastroenteritis
- Urinary tract infection/pyelonephritis, kidney stones
- Gynecological: ectopic pregnancy, ovarian torsion, PID

Chronic/Recurrent Causes

- GERD, peptic ulcer disease
- IBS
- Inflammatory bowel disease
- Chronic constipation
- Chronic pancreatitis
- Gynecological: endometriosis, ovarian cysts
- Malignancy

What to Do in the Office

1. Rapid Initial Assessment

- Vitals: BP, HR, RR, SpO_2, temperature.
- Observe for shock: hypotension, tachycardia, altered LOC.
- Look for peritonitis: rigidity, rebound, guarding.

2. Focused History

- Onset, location, radiation, character, severity.
- Timing: acute vs chronic, continuous vs intermittent.
- Associated symptoms: fever, vomiting, diarrhea, hematemesis, melena, hematochezia, dysuria, vaginal bleeding/discharge.

- Past history: surgeries, GI disease, gynecological history.

3. Focused Exam

- General: appearance, hydration, jaundice, pallor.
- Abdomen: inspection, bowel sounds, palpation (tenderness, peritonitis, organomegaly).
- Rectal exam: if GI bleed or obstruction suspected.
- Pelvic exam: if gynecological cause possible.

4. In-Office Investigations (if available)

- Urinalysis ± urine culture.
- Urine pregnancy test (all women of reproductive age).
- CBC, electrolytes, LFTs, amylase/lipase (if office phlebotomy available, otherwise refer).
- ECG (if epigastric pain, rule out cardiac cause).

5. Initial Management in Office

- Keep NPO if acute abdomen suspected.
- Analgesia (acetaminophen, NSAIDs if safe; avoid strong opioids before surgical consult).
- Antiemetics if vomiting.

- Antibiotics if strong suspicion of intra-abdominal infection and immediate hospital transfer.

When to Refer to ED (Urgent)

- Hemodynamic instability, shock.
- Signs of peritonitis (rebound, rigidity, guarding).
- GI bleed (hematemesis, melena, hematochezia with instability).
- Suspected surgical emergencies: appendicitis, bowel obstruction, perforation, ectopic pregnancy, ovarian torsion.
- Severe pancreatitis.

When to Refer to Specialists (Non-Urgent)

- **Gastroenterology:** IBD, peptic ulcer disease, chronic unexplained abdominal pain, GI malignancy suspicion.
- **Gynecology:** endometriosis, ovarian cysts, chronic pelvic pain.
- **General surgery:** recurrent biliary colic, elective hernia repair.
- **Urology:** recurrent kidney stones.

When to Manage in Primary Care

- Gastroenteritis (mild, self-limiting).
- Constipation.
- Mild GERD, dyspepsia.
- Irritable bowel syndrome.
- Stable chronic conditions with follow-up (functional abdominal pain, post-infectious pain).

Pocket Box – Office Abdominal Pain Quick Reference

- **Step 1:** Vitals → look for instability/shock.
- **Step 2:** Focused history + exam (red flags: peritonitis, bleeding, pregnancy).
- **Step 3:**
  - **Unstable/red flag:** NPO → IV access if possible → EMS transfer.
  - **Stable:** Urinalysis, pregnancy test, ECG (if epigastric), labs/imaging as outpatient.
- **Step 4:** Manage benign conditions in office; refer GI/Gyn/Surgery as indicated.

8. Headache (acute and chronic)

Introduction

Headache is a frequent complaint in family medicine. While most are benign (tension, migraine), some represent life-threatening emergencies. The family physician must quickly recognize red flags, manage common primary headaches in the office, and know when urgent referral is required.

Differential Diagnosis

Primary Headaches

- Tension-type headache
- Migraine (with or without aura)
- Cluster headache

Secondary Headaches (serious)

- Subarachnoid hemorrhage (thunderclap headache)
- Intracranial hemorrhage (trauma, aneurysm, AVM)
- Meningitis/encephalitis

- Temporal arteritis (age >50, scalp tenderness, vision changes)
- Brain tumour (progressive, new neuro deficits, raised ICP signs)

Secondary Headaches (benign or common)

- Sinusitis
- Medication overuse headache
- Cervical spine disease
- Hypertension (usually severe, malignant)

What to Do in the Office

1. Rapid Initial Assessment

- Check vitals, including BP and temperature.
- Assess for red flags: sudden severe headache, fever/neck stiffness, neuro deficits, altered LOC.

2. Focused History

- Onset: sudden vs gradual.
- Duration and frequency.
- Character: throbbing, pressure, unilateral vs bilateral.
- Associated symptoms: nausea, vomiting, photophobia, aura, weakness, vision changes.

- Past history: migraines, trauma, risk factors for vascular disease.

3. Focused Exam

- Neuro exam: cranial nerves, motor, reflexes, coordination.
- Fundoscopy: papilledema.
- Neck stiffness (meningitis, SAH).
- Temporal artery tenderness in older patients.
- ENT/sinus exam.

4. In-Office Investigations (if available)

- ESR/CRP in suspected temporal arteritis.
- Glucose, BP check (exclude metabolic cause or hypertensive emergency).
- Imaging (CT/MRI) is not done in-office — arrange urgently if red flags.

5. Initial Management in Office

- **Migraine:** NSAIDs, acetaminophen, or triptans (if no contraindications). Antiemetic if nausea.
- **Tension headache:** NSAIDs/acetaminophen, reassurance, lifestyle modification (stress, posture, sleep).
- **Cluster headache:** Refer to ED/specialist for O_2 and triptan therapy.

- **Suspected temporal arteritis:** Start high-dose steroids immediately, urgent referral for biopsy.

When to Refer to ED (Urgent)

- Sudden "thunderclap" headache (rule out SAH).
- New headache with fever, neck stiffness, altered mental status (suspect meningitis/encephalitis).
- Headache with focal neuro deficits, seizure, or papilledema.
- Headache post-trauma with neuro change.
- Hypertensive emergency with severe headache.

When to Refer to Specialists (Non-Urgent)

- **Neurology:** frequent disabling migraines not controlled with first-line therapy, cluster headaches, chronic daily headache, atypical headache syndromes.
- **Ophthalmology:** vision changes, papilledema, suspected glaucoma.
- **ENT:** chronic sinus-related headaches.

When to Manage in Primary Care

- Stable tension-type headaches.
- Migraines responsive to first-line treatment.
- Sinusitis-related headaches.
- Medication overuse headaches (by adjusting/withdrawing offending drugs).

Pocket Box – Office Headache Quick Reference

- **Step 1:** Vitals, neuro exam, check red flags.
- **Step 2:**
  - **Red flags present:** EMS transfer or urgent imaging referral.
  - **No red flags:** Treat as migraine, tension, or sinus-related.
- **Step 3:** ESR/CRP if >50 with temporal tenderness/vision symptoms → start steroids, urgent referral.
- **Step 4:** Specialist referral if recurrent, disabling, or atypical.

9. Back Pain

Introduction

Back pain is one of the most common reasons for visits to family physicians. While most cases are benign and mechanical, some are associated with serious underlying pathology. The challenge in primary care is to identify red flags that require urgent investigation or referral, while managing the majority conservatively in the office.

Differential Diagnosis

Mechanical/Benign

- Lumbar strain, sprain
- Degenerative disc disease, osteoarthritis
- Spondylosis, spondylolisthesis
- Postural or occupational strain

Neurological

- Herniated disc with radiculopathy
- Spinal stenosis
- Cauda equina syndrome (emergency)

Infectious/Inflammatory

- Vertebral osteomyelitis/discitis
- Epidural abscess
- Ankylosing spondylitis, other spondyloarthropathies

Malignant

- Spinal metastases (breast, prostate, lung, renal, thyroid)
- Primary bone malignancy (rare)

Other Causes

- Kidney stones, pyelonephritis
- Abdominal aortic aneurysm (AAA)
- Pancreatitis

What to Do in the Office

1. Rapid Initial Assessment

- Vitals: fever, hypotension, tachycardia.
- Screen for red flags: neuro deficits, bowel/bladder involvement, trauma, cancer history, infection risk.

2. Focused History

- Onset: sudden vs gradual.
- Character: localized vs radicular, constant vs intermittent.
- Aggravating/relieving factors.

- Associated symptoms: leg weakness, saddle anesthesia, urinary retention/incontinence, fever, weight loss, night sweats.
- Past history: cancer, immunosuppression, trauma, IV drug use.

3. Focused Exam

- Inspect posture, gait.
- Palpate spine for tenderness.
- Neuro exam: strength, reflexes, sensation in lower limbs.
- Straight leg raise (disc herniation).
- Abdominal exam (exclude AAA, renal causes).

4. In-Office Investigations (if available)

- Urinalysis (if renal cause suspected).
- ESR/CRP if infection or malignancy suspected.
- Imaging not required for acute nonspecific back pain (<6 weeks, no red flags).
- Arrange urgent imaging (X-ray, MRI) if red flags present.

5. Initial Management in Office

- Analgesia: acetaminophen, NSAIDs first-line.

- Encourage activity and early mobilization (avoid bed rest).
- Physiotherapy referral for mechanical back pain.
- Heat, stretching, ergonomics advice.
- Short course of muscle relaxants if severe spasm.

When to Refer to ED (Urgent)

- Cauda equina syndrome (urinary retention/incontinence, saddle anesthesia, bilateral leg weakness).
- Severe or progressive neurological deficit.
- Suspected epidural abscess (fever, spinal tenderness, neuro symptoms).
- Severe trauma with unstable spine suspicion.
- Suspected AAA rupture.

When to Refer to Specialists (Non-Urgent)

- **Orthopedics/Neurosurgery:** persistent radiculopathy, spinal stenosis, herniated disc not improving after 6–8 weeks conservative therapy.

- **Rheumatology:** inflammatory back pain (young patient, morning stiffness, improved with exercise).
- **Oncology:** suspicion of metastatic disease.
- **Physiatry/Chronic pain:** persistent pain despite conservative measures.

When to Manage in Primary Care

- Acute nonspecific mechanical back pain (<6 weeks, no red flags).
- Recurrent mechanical strain with lifestyle/occupational triggers.
- Stable chronic low back pain responding to physiotherapy and analgesia.
- Mild radiculopathy improving with conservative therapy.

Pocket Box – Office Back Pain Quick Reference

- **Step 1:** Vitals, screen for red flags (neuro deficits, cancer, infection, trauma, AAA).
- **Step 2:**
    - **Red flags present:** urgent imaging + EMS transfer or ED referral.

- **No red flags:** reassure, analgesia, encourage activity, physio referral.
- **Step 3:**
  - Reassess if persistent >6 weeks, worsening, or new neuro symptoms.
  - Non-urgent referral to ortho/rheum/pain clinic if needed.

10. Fatigue

Introduction

Fatigue is a common and often nonspecific complaint in family practice. It may be related to lifestyle factors, psychological conditions, chronic disease, or serious systemic illness. The challenge in primary care is to identify reversible or dangerous causes while avoiding unnecessary investigations.

Differential Diagnosis

Lifestyle/Functional

- Poor sleep (insomnia, shift work)
- Deconditioning, overwork
- Poor diet, sedentary lifestyle

Psychological

- Depression
- Anxiety
- Chronic stress, burnout

Endocrine/Metabolic

- Hypothyroidism

- Diabetes (poorly controlled, undiagnosed)
- Adrenal insufficiency

Hematologic/Nutritional

- Anemia (iron deficiency, chronic disease, B12/folate deficiency)
- Malnutrition, vitamin D deficiency

Infectious

- Viral infections (EBV, CMV, HIV, hepatitis)
- Chronic infections (TB, endocarditis)

Other Systemic

- Chronic kidney disease
- Liver disease
- Malignancy

What to Do in the Office

1. Initial Assessment

- Vitals: BP, HR, temperature, weight, BMI.
- General appearance: pallor, jaundice, cachexia, lymphadenopathy.

2. Focused History

- Onset, duration (acute vs chronic).
- Sleep quality, occupation, activity level.
- Psychological symptoms (low mood, anxiety, anhedonia).
- Red flags: unintentional weight loss, night sweats, fever, bleeding/bruising.
- Medications (sedatives, antihistamines, beta-blockers).

3. Focused Exam

- General: pallor, thyroid exam, lymph nodes, hepatosplenomegaly.
- Neuro: reflexes (hypothyroidism, B12 deficiency).
- Cardiac/respiratory: murmurs, signs of heart failure.

4. In-Office Investigations (initial screening)

- CBC (anemia, infection).
- TSH (thyroid disease).
- Fasting glucose or HbA1c (diabetes).
- Ferritin, B12, folate (nutritional).
- Renal and liver function tests.
- ESR/CRP if systemic illness suspected.

5. Initial Management in Office

- Address lifestyle contributors (sleep hygiene, exercise, diet).

- Treat underlying conditions (iron supplementation, thyroid replacement, diabetes optimization).
- Screen and manage depression/anxiety.
- Arrange follow-up to review labs and progress.

When to Refer to ED (Urgent)

- Severe anemia with hemodynamic instability.
- Fever, night sweats, weight loss with suspected malignancy or sepsis.
- New neurological deficits (e.g., weakness, ataxia with B12 deficiency).

When to Refer to Specialists (Non-Urgent)

- **Endocrinology:** unclear thyroid/adrenal/metabolic cause.
- **Hematology:** unexplained anemia, abnormal blood film.
- **Psychiatry:** severe depression, suicidality, or complex psychiatric fatigue.
- **Oncology/Internal Medicine:** suspicion of malignancy after initial work-up.

When to Manage in Primary Care

- Fatigue due to lifestyle causes, stress, or mild depression/anxiety.
- Stable chronic conditions (treated hypothyroidism, well-controlled diabetes).
- Nutritional deficiencies (iron, B12, vitamin D).
- Post-viral fatigue with gradual improvement.

Pocket Box – Office Fatigue Quick Reference

- **Step 1:** Vitals, general inspection.
- **Step 2:** History → sleep, mood, red flags (fever, weight loss, night sweats).
- **Step 3:** Exam → thyroid, lymph nodes, pallor, neuro signs.
- **Step 4:** Labs → CBC, TSH, HbA1c, ferritin, B12/folate, renal/liver function.
- **Step 5:**
    - **Red flags present:** urgent referral/ED.
    - **No red flags:** treat lifestyle/psychological/nutritional causes, follow up.

11. Dizziness & Vertigo

Introduction

Dizziness is a vague but common complaint in family practice. It may be described as lightheadedness, imbalance, presyncope, or true spinning vertigo. The role of the family physician is to clarify what the patient means, rule out life-threatening or neurologic causes, and manage common benign conditions such as BPPV (benign paroxysmal positional vertigo).

Differential Diagnosis

Vertigo (spinning sensation)

- **Peripheral:**
    - Benign paroxysmal positional vertigo (BPPV)
    - Vestibular neuritis
    - Ménière's disease
    - Acute otitis media/labyrinthitis
- **Central:**
    - Stroke (posterior circulation)
    - Multiple sclerosis
    - Brain tumour

Non-vertiginous dizziness

- Presyncope: arrhythmia, orthostatic hypotension, anemia.
- Disequilibrium: Parkinson's disease, neuropathy, musculoskeletal disorders.
- Psychiatric: anxiety, panic attacks.

What to Do in the Office

1. Rapid Initial Assessment

- Vitals: BP (including orthostatic), HR, RR, O_2 sat.
- Assess for acute neurological symptoms: ataxia, diplopia, dysarthria, weakness.

2. Focused History

- Clarify: spinning vs lightheadedness vs imbalance.
- Onset and triggers (sudden, positional, continuous).
- Duration of episodes (seconds vs hours vs persistent).
- Associated symptoms: nausea, vomiting, hearing loss, tinnitus, chest pain, palpitations.
- Past history: cardiovascular disease, stroke risk factors, ear disease.

3. Focused Exam

- Neurological: cranial nerves, coordination, gait, Romberg test.
- HINTS exam (head impulse, nystagmus, test of skew) if acute vertigo.
- ENT: ear canal, tympanic membrane.
- Cardiovascular: auscultation, rhythm, orthostatic vitals.

4. In-Office Investigations (if available)

- ECG (rule out arrhythmia).
- CBC if anemia suspected.
- Glucose (hypoglycemia).

5. Initial Management in Office

- **BPPV:** Epley maneuver, reassurance.
- **Vestibular neuritis/labyrinthitis:** short course vestibular suppressants (meclizine, dimenhydrinate), steroids sometimes used.
- **Ménière's disease:** salt restriction, diuretics, ENT referral.
- **Orthostatic hypotension:** hydration, review medications.
- **Anxiety-related:** reassurance, CBT referral, consider SSRI if persistent.

When to Refer to ED (Urgent)

- Acute vertigo with neurological deficits (suspected stroke/TIA).
- Severe, continuous vertigo not improving.
- Hemodynamic instability (arrhythmia, severe hypotension).
- Syncope or collapse.

When to Refer to Specialists (Non-Urgent)

- **ENT/Neurology:** persistent or recurrent vertigo (BPPV not resolving, Ménière's disease).
- **Cardiology:** recurrent presyncope/syncope with abnormal ECG or arrhythmia.
- **Neurology:** suspected MS, unexplained disequilibrium.

When to Manage in Primary Care

- Typical BPPV responding to repositioning maneuvers.
- Mild, self-limited viral labyrinthitis.
- Orthostatic hypotension due to dehydration or meds (review and adjust).
- Anxiety-related dizziness with reassurance and follow-up.

Pocket Box – Office Dizziness & Vertigo Quick Reference

- **Step 1:** Vitals (orthostatic), clarify type (vertigo vs presyncope vs imbalance).
- **Step 2:**
    - **Red flags:** neuro deficits, continuous severe vertigo, arrhythmia → ED transfer.
    - **No red flags:** focused ENT/neuro exam, ECG, labs if indicated.
- **Step 3:**
    - **Likely BPPV:** perform Epley maneuver.
    - **Infectious/viral:** short-term vestibular suppressant, supportive care.
    - **Orthostatic/anxiety:** treat underlying cause.
- **Step 4:** Refer ENT/Neuro/Cardiology if persistent, recurrent, or unexplained.

12. Rash & Skin Lesions

Introduction

Rashes and skin lesions are frequent in family medicine, ranging from mild allergic reactions to life-threatening dermatologic emergencies. Many can be diagnosed clinically in the office, but some require urgent referral. A structured approach to morphology, distribution, and associated systemic features helps guide diagnosis and management.

Differential Diagnosis

Infectious

- Bacterial: cellulitis, impetigo, erysipelas
- Viral: varicella, herpes zoster, viral exanthems
- Fungal: tinea corporis, candidiasis
- Parasitic: scabies, lice

Inflammatory/Allergic

- Eczema (atopic dermatitis)
- Psoriasis
- Urticaria (hives)

- Contact dermatitis (irritant, allergic, e.g. Poison Ivy)
- Drug eruptions

Malignant/Precancerous

- Basal cell carcinoma (BCC)
- Squamous cell carcinoma (SCC)
- Melanoma
- Actinic keratosis

Serious Emergencies

- Stevens-Johnson syndrome (SJS) / Toxic epidermal necrolysis (TEN)
- Meningococcemia (purpura, systemic illness)
- Necrotizing fasciitis

What to Do in the Office

1. Initial Assessment

- Vitals (fever, hypotension, tachycardia).
- Assess for systemic toxicity: malaise, hypotension, confusion.
- Morphology: macule, papule, vesicle, pustule, plaque, nodule.
- Distribution: localized vs generalized, symmetrical vs asymmetrical.

2. Focused History

- Onset and progression (sudden vs gradual).
- Itching, pain, burning, systemic symptoms.
- Recent infections, new medications, allergens, exposures.
- Past history: eczema, psoriasis, skin cancer, immunosuppression.

3. Focused Exam

- Full skin inspection (don't forget scalp, nails, mucous membranes).
- Palpation for warmth, induration, tenderness.
- Check for lymphadenopathy.
- Document lesion size, shape, borders, color.

4. In-Office Investigations

- Usually clinical diagnosis.
- KOH prep if fungal suspected.
- Bacterial culture from pustule/ulcer if needed.
- Dermoscopy if available for pigmented lesions.

5. Initial Management

- **Mild eczema/contact dermatitis:** topical steroids, emollients, avoid triggers.
- **Urticaria:** antihistamines, identify allergens.
- **Cellulitis (mild):** oral antibiotics, close follow-up.
- **Tinea/candidiasis:** topical antifungals.
- **Suspicious lesion:** biopsy or urgent referral.

When to Refer to ED (Urgent)

- Rash with systemic toxicity (fever, hypotension, altered LOC).
- Suspected meningococcemia (fever + purpura).
- Severe blistering/drug reaction (SJS/TEN).
- Necrotizing fasciitis (pain out of proportion, rapidly spreading erythema, crepitus).

When to Refer to Specialists (Non-Urgent)

- **Dermatology:** uncertain pigmented lesion (r/o melanoma), chronic/refractory eczema or psoriasis, recurrent allergic/contact dermatitis.

- **Oncology/Dermatology:** confirmed or suspected skin cancer.
- **Allergy/Immunology:** recurrent urticaria, severe allergic skin conditions.

When to Manage in Primary Care

- Mild eczema, psoriasis, acne.
- Viral exanthems, localized fungal infections.
- Mild urticaria, contact dermatitis (Poison Ivy, irritants).
- Uncomplicated cellulitis responsive to oral antibiotics.

Pocket Box – Office Rash & Skin Lesions Quick Reference

- **Step 1:** Vitals, assess systemic illness.
- **Step 2:** History → onset, meds, exposures, systemic symptoms.
- **Step 3:** Exam → morphology, distribution, mucous membranes.
- **Step 4:**
    - **Red flags present:** meningococcemia, SJS/TEN, nec fasc → EMS transfer.

- o **No red flags:** treat common causes (eczema, fungal, cellulitis, urticaria).
- **Step 5:** Refer dermatology for uncertain pigmented lesions, refractory conditions, or suspected malignancy.

13. Fever of Unknown Origin

Introduction

Fever of unknown origin (FUO) is defined as fever >38.3°C on several occasions, lasting more than 3 weeks, with no diagnosis after initial evaluation. In family practice, most fevers are due to self-limited infections, but persistent or unexplained fevers require systematic evaluation. The family physician's role is to rule out common and serious causes, initiate initial investigations, and identify when urgent referral is required.

Differential Diagnosis

Infectious

- Tuberculosis
- Endocarditis
- Abscess (occult intra-abdominal, dental, pelvic)
- HIV and other chronic viral infections

Inflammatory/Autoimmune

- Giant cell arteritis / polymyalgia rheumatica
- Systemic lupus erythematosus (SLE)

- Rheumatoid arthritis, vasculitis

Malignancy

- Lymphoma, leukemia
- Renal cell carcinoma
- Hepatocellular carcinoma

Miscellaneous

- Drug fever
- Factitious fever
- Endocrine disorders (thyroiditis, adrenal insufficiency)

What to Do in the Office

1. Initial Assessment

- Vitals: temperature (document pattern), BP, HR, SpO$_2$.
- General appearance: weight loss, night sweats, cachexia, pallor.

2. Focused History

- Onset, duration, fever pattern (daily, intermittent).
- Associated symptoms: night sweats, weight loss, cough, dysuria, abdominal pain, rash, joint pain.

- Past medical history: TB exposure, prosthetic valves, autoimmune disease, malignancy.
- Travel history, pets/animal exposure, occupational risks.
- Medications (drug fever).

3. Focused Exam

- General: lymphadenopathy, hepatosplenomegaly.
- Heart: murmurs (endocarditis).
- Chest: crackles, consolidation.
- Abdomen: tenderness, organomegaly, masses.
- Skin: rashes, lesions, stigmata of endocarditis.
- Joints: swelling, stiffness, tenderness.

4. In-Office Investigations (initial screen)

- CBC with differential.
- ESR, CRP.
- Blood cultures (x2–3, if available).
- Urinalysis ± urine culture.
- Chest X-ray.
- HIV, TB testing if risk factors present.
- Basic metabolic panel, LFTs.

5. Initial Management in Office

- Most stable patients → outpatient work-up and follow-up.

- Symptomatic treatment (hydration, antipyretics).
- Avoid empiric antibiotics unless patient is unstable or septic.

When to Refer to ED (Urgent)

- Hemodynamic instability, sepsis.
- Immunocompromised patient with persistent fever.
- Neurological symptoms with fever (meningitis, encephalitis).
- FUO with rapid deterioration, severe weight loss, or respiratory compromise.

When to Refer to Specialists (Non-Urgent)

- **Infectious Diseases:** persistent unexplained fever, suspected TB, endocarditis, HIV.
- **Rheumatology:** suspected autoimmune/vasculitis cause.
- **Oncology/Hematology:** suspected malignancy (abnormal blood counts, lymphadenopathy, B symptoms).

When to Manage in Primary Care

- Self-limited viral infections with short duration.
- Low-grade fever associated with minor localized infections (sinusitis, dental abscess) with clear source.
- Patients improving clinically with supportive care and negative red flags.

Pocket Box – Office FUO Quick Reference

- **Step 1:** Confirm fever pattern, check vitals.
- **Step 2:** History → exposures, travel, systemic symptoms.
- **Step 3:** Exam → lymph nodes, murmurs, abdomen, skin, joints.
- **Step 4:** Initial work-up → CBC, ESR/CRP, blood/urine cultures, CXR.
- **Step 5:**
    - **Unstable/septic:** EMS transfer to ED.
    - **Stable, no red flags:** outpatient work-up + follow-up.
    - **Suspicion of TB/autoimmune/malignanc

> **y:** refer ID, rheumatology, oncology.

14. Depression, Anxiety & Insomnia

Introduction

Mental health concerns are among the most common issues managed in family practice. Depression, anxiety, and insomnia often present together and significantly impact quality of life, physical health, and function. Family physicians play a central role in early detection, diagnosis, initial management, and referral when higher-level care is needed.

Differential Diagnosis

Depression

- Major depressive disorder
- Adjustment disorder with depressed mood
- Bipolar disorder (screen before starting antidepressants)
- Dysthymia (persistent depressive disorder)

Anxiety

- Generalized anxiety disorder (GAD)

- Panic disorder
- Social anxiety disorder
- PTSD, OCD (screen and refer if suspected)

Insomnia

- Primary insomnia
- Secondary to depression/anxiety
- Substance-related (alcohol, caffeine, stimulants)
- Medical conditions: chronic pain, sleep apnea, restless leg syndrome

Other Causes to Exclude

- Thyroid disease
- Anemia
- Chronic medical illness
- Medication-induced (beta-blockers, corticosteroids, stimulants)

What to Do in the Office

1. Initial Assessment

- Vitals, BMI.
- Screen for substance use (alcohol, drugs, caffeine).
- Screen for suicide risk: passive/active ideation, plan, means, protective factors.

2. Focused History

- Duration, severity, functional impairment.
- Associated symptoms: sleep disturbance, appetite/weight change, fatigue, irritability.
- Past psychiatric history, family history.
- Stressors, supports, coping strategies.

3. Focused Exam

- Mental status exam: appearance, mood, affect, thought process, cognition.
- Rule out medical contributors (thyroid exam, neuro exam if indicated).

4. In-Office Investigations

- CBC, TSH, glucose if medical contributors suspected.
- Standardized tools: PHQ-9 (depression), GAD-7 (anxiety), Insomnia Severity Index.

5. Initial Management in Office

- Psychoeducation: normalize discussion of mental health.
- Lifestyle: sleep hygiene, exercise, limit caffeine/alcohol.
- **Mild depression/anxiety:** counseling, CBT referral, guided self-help.

- **Moderate-severe:** consider SSRIs/SNRIs, close follow-up.
- **Insomnia:** behavioral therapy first-line, short-term sleep aids only if severe.
- Safety planning if suicidal thoughts (remove means, crisis numbers, family involvement).

When to Refer to ED (Urgent)

- Active suicidal ideation with plan/intent.
- Severe self-neglect, inability to care for self.
- Psychotic depression or mania.
- Acute risk of harm to self or others.

When to Refer to Specialists (Non-Urgent)

- **Psychiatry:**
    - Treatment-resistant depression or anxiety.
    - Bipolar disorder or suspected psychotic features.
    - Severe OCD, PTSD.
- **Sleep medicine:** refractory insomnia, suspected sleep apnea.

- **Psychology/CBT programs:** for ongoing therapy.

When to Manage in Primary Care

- Mild to moderate depression and anxiety responding to first-line therapy.
- Insomnia improved with sleep hygiene, short-term pharmacotherapy, or CBT-I.
- Stable patients without red flags, managed with regular follow-up.

Pocket Box – Office Depression, Anxiety & Insomnia Quick Reference

- **Step 1:** Screen for depression (PHQ-9), anxiety (GAD-7), suicide risk.
- **Step 2:** Rule out medical causes (TSH, CBC, meds, chronic illness).
- **Step 3:**
    - **Red flags:** suicidality, psychosis, mania → ED referral.
    - **No red flags:** start lifestyle, CBT, consider SSRI/SNRI.

- **Step 4:** Follow up in 2–4 weeks for med initiation, sooner if safety concerns.
- **Step 5:** Refer psychiatry if treatment-resistant, severe, or unclear diagnosis.

15. Pediatric Presentations

Introduction

Children frequently present to family physicians with acute and chronic concerns. Most conditions are benign and self-limiting, but the challenge is identifying red flags that may indicate serious illness. Pediatric assessment in the office relies heavily on careful history, physical exam, growth and development monitoring, and knowing when to escalate to emergency or specialty care.

Differential Diagnosis by Symptom

Fever

- Viral infection (most common)
- Bacterial infection: otitis media, strep throat, UTI, pneumonia
- Serious: sepsis, meningitis, Kawasaki disease

Vomiting

- Gastroenteritis (most common)
- UTI
- Increased intracranial pressure (head trauma, tumor, hydrocephalus)

- GI obstruction (pyloric stenosis, intussusception, malrotation)

Cough/Wheeze

- Viral URTI, bronchiolitis
- Asthma
- Pneumonia
- Foreign body aspiration

Developmental Delay

- Global developmental delay (genetic, metabolic, neurologic)
- Isolated delay: speech/language, motor, social
- Autism spectrum disorder
- Environmental factors: neglect, limited stimulation

What to Do in the Office

1. Initial Assessment

- Vitals: HR, RR, SpO_2, temperature (age-appropriate norms).
- Growth chart review (weight, height, head circumference).
- General appearance: alert vs lethargic, hydration status, interaction with caregiver.

2. Focused History

- Symptom onset, duration, severity.
- Feeding, urine/stool output.
- Immunization status.
- Sick contacts, recent travel.
- Developmental milestones (gross motor, fine motor, language, social).

3. Focused Exam

- Full physical exam (HEENT, chest, abdomen, neuro).
- Respiratory distress signs: retractions, nasal flaring, grunting.
- Neuro: tone, reflexes, responsiveness.
- Skin: rashes, dehydration signs, bruising.

4. In-Office Investigations (if available)

- Urinalysis ± urine culture for febrile child <2 years.
- Rapid strep test if pharyngitis suspected.
- Pulse oximetry for respiratory symptoms.
- Basic bloodwork if systemic illness suspected (often arranged via ED).

5. Initial Management in Office

- **Fever:** antipyretics (acetaminophen, ibuprofen if >6 months), fluids.

- **Vomiting:** oral rehydration solution (ORS), ondansetron if persistent.
- **Cough/wheeze:** salbutamol trial if asthma suspected, oxygen if hypoxic.
- **Developmental delay:** counsel parents, initiate referrals (speech therapy, developmental pediatrics, audiology).

When to Refer to ED (Urgent)

- Lethargy, poor perfusion, unresponsiveness.
- Persistent vomiting with dehydration or bilious emesis.
- Respiratory distress, hypoxia (SpO_2 <90%).
- Suspected meningitis, sepsis, Kawasaki disease.
- Seizures or acute neurological change.
- Signs of intestinal obstruction (projectile vomiting, bloody stools, abdominal distension).

When to Refer to Specialists (Non-Urgent)

- **Pediatrics:** recurrent infections, complex chronic conditions, unclear diagnosis.
- **Respirology:** asthma not controlled on first-line therapy.

- **Developmental Pediatrics/Child Psych:** developmental delay, suspected autism.
- **Neurology:** seizures, motor delay with abnormal neuro exam.
- **ENT/Audiology:** speech delay with possible hearing impairment.

When to Manage in Primary Care

- Viral URTI, viral gastroenteritis.
- Mild wheeze responsive to bronchodilator.
- Simple otitis media, pharyngitis, mild pneumonia.
- Mild febrile illness in well-appearing child.
- Developmental variations within normal range, monitored with anticipatory guidance.

Pocket Box – Office Pediatric Quick Reference

- **Step 1:** Vitals + growth chart + overall appearance.
- **Step 2:**
    - Fever: UTI screen, hydration, antipyretics.

- - Vomiting: hydration, r/o obstruction, ORS.
  - Cough/wheeze: O_2, salbutamol trial, CXR if pneumonia suspected.
  - Developmental delay: milestone review, early referral.
- **Step 3:**
  - **Red flags:** lethargy, hypoxia, bilious vomiting, neuro deficits → ED transfer.

No red flags: treat in office, follow closely, refer specialists as needed.

16. Geriatric Presentations

Introduction

Older adults often present with nonspecific or overlapping complaints. Falls, confusion, mobility issues, and polypharmacy are among the most common reasons for consultation. In family medicine, the physician's role is to identify acute emergencies, address reversible contributors, optimize chronic care, and coordinate multidisciplinary support.

Differential Diagnosis

Falls

- Mechanical fall (environmental, tripping, poor vision)
- Neurological: stroke, Parkinson's, peripheral neuropathy
- Cardiovascular: syncope, arrhythmias, orthostatic hypotension
- Musculoskeletal: arthritis, frailty, sarcopenia
- Medications (sedatives, antihypertensives, hypoglycemics)

Confusion (Delirium vs Dementia)

- Delirium (infection, dehydration, medication, metabolic causes)
- Dementia (Alzheimer's, vascular, Lewy body, frontotemporal)
- Depression ("pseudodementia")
- Stroke/TIA

Mobility Issues

- Osteoarthritis, osteoporosis with fractures
- Neurologic disease (Parkinson's, stroke sequelae, neuropathy)
- Frailty/deconditioning

Polypharmacy

- Drug–drug interactions
- Adverse drug effects (falls, delirium, renal/hepatic impairment)
- Inappropriate prescribing (Beers Criteria)

What to Do in the Office

1. Initial Assessment

- Vitals including orthostatic BP.
- General appearance: hydration, gait, frailty, nutrition.
- Screen cognition (MMSE, MoCA) and mood (GDS).

- Review medication list carefully.

2. Focused History

- For falls: circumstances, preceding symptoms (dizziness, syncope), frequency.
- For confusion: onset (acute vs chronic), progression, associated infection or drug changes.
- For mobility: pain, stiffness, neurologic symptoms, ADL limitations.
- For polypharmacy: indication for each drug, adherence, adverse effects.

3. Focused Exam

- Neuro: motor, sensation, reflexes, balance, gait assessment (Timed Up and Go).
- MSK: joint tenderness, ROM, muscle strength.
- CVS: murmurs, arrhythmias, postural vitals.
- Mental status: orientation, attention, recall.

4. In-Office Investigations (initial)

- CBC, electrolytes, renal/liver function (confusion, frailty, drug monitoring).
- Urinalysis if delirium suspected.
- ECG if arrhythmia/syncope suspected.
- Vitamin B12, TSH (if confusion).

- Medication review (include OTC/herbals).

5. Initial Management in Office

- **Falls:** address hazards, correct vision/hearing, physiotherapy referral, walking aids.
- **Confusion:** treat reversible causes (infection, dehydration, med side effects).
- **Mobility:** analgesia, physio, exercise, osteoporosis screening.
- **Polypharmacy:** deprescribe unnecessary meds, simplify regimen, adjust doses.

When to Refer to ED (Urgent)

- Falls with serious injury (hip fracture, head trauma).
- Acute delirium with hemodynamic instability, sepsis, or stroke suspicion.
- Syncope with arrhythmia or cardiac cause suspected.
- New focal neurological deficits.

When to Refer to Specialists (Non-Urgent)

- **Geriatrics:** complex multimorbidity, frailty, recurrent falls, polypharmacy.
- **Neurology:** Parkinson's disease, atypical dementias, unexplained recurrent falls.
- **Orthopedics:** fractures, severe osteoarthritis requiring surgery.
- **Psychiatry:** severe depression, behavioral symptoms in dementia.

When to Manage in Primary Care

- Stable mild dementia with caregiver support.
- Mild osteoarthritis with conservative management.
- Frailty management with nutrition, exercise, fall prevention.
- Medication review and deprescribing.

Pocket Box – Office Geriatric Quick Reference

- **Step 1:** Vitals, cognition screen, medication review.
- **Step 2:**
  - Falls → assess cause (neuro, cardio, MSK, meds, environment).

- Confusion → acute (delirium) vs chronic (dementia).
- Mobility → MSK vs neuro vs frailty.
- Polypharmacy → review & deprescribe.
- **Step 3:**
  - **Red flags:** fracture, acute delirium, stroke, syncope → ED.

Stable: treat reversible causes, arrange follow-up, refer geriatric/rehab if needed.

Part III – Clinical Systems

This page has been left intentionally blank

Section 1: Cardiovascular Medicine

17. Hypertension

Diagnosis

- Office BP: ≥140/90 (average of 2–3 visits, proper technique).
- Home BP: ≥135/85.
- Ambulatory (24-hr): ≥130/80.
- Confirm with home/ambulatory monitoring if possible.

Differential Diagnosis

- **Primary (essential HTN):** majority.
- **Secondary:** CKD, renovascular disease, hyperaldosteronism, pheochromocytoma, thyroid disease, Cushing's, sleep apnea, meds (NSAIDs, OCPs, steroids, stimulants).

Initial Office Work-Up

- Labs: CBC, electrolytes, creatinine/eGFR, glucose/HbA1c, lipids, urinalysis.
- ECG for LVH/arrhythmias/ischemia.

- Assess for end-organ damage: fundoscopy, neuro, renal, cardiac.

Lifestyle Management (all patients)

- Weight control (BMI 18.5–24.9).
- DASH diet, low sodium (<2000 mg/day).
- Exercise (150 min/week).
- Alcohol moderation, smoking cessation, stress management.

Pharmacologic Therapy

- Start if:
    - Persistent BP ≥140/90, OR
    - Diabetes, CKD, ASCVD, organ damage, OR
    - Severe HTN ≥180/110.
- First-line: thiazide/thiazide-like, ACEi/ARB, CCB.
- Beta-blocker if CAD, post-MI, or specific indication.
- Combination therapy often needed.
- Targets: <140/90 (most), <130/80 (diabetes, CKD, high CV risk).

Follow-Up

- Reassess BP: 1–2 months after med changes.
- Monitor electrolytes/renal function with ACEi/ARB/diuretics.
- Annual review for complications + adherence.

Referral

- **ED (urgent):** hypertensive emergency (>180/120 with organ damage), hypertensive urgency with symptoms.
- **Specialist (non-urgent):**
  - Nephrology: resistant HTN (≥3 meds including diuretic).
  - Endocrinology: suspected secondary cause.
  - Cardiology: comorbid IHD, HF, LVH.

Primary Care Management

- Most uncomplicated essential HTN.
- Controlled patients on 1–3 meds.
- Long-term monitoring + lifestyle counseling.

18. Dyslipidemia & ASCVD Prevention

Screening & Diagnosis

- Screen adults ≥40 years, earlier if high risk (diabetes, family history, CKD, hypertension).
- Labs: fasting or non-fasting lipid panel (TC, LDL-C, HDL-C, TG).
- Calculate 10-year ASCVD risk (e.g., Framingham Risk Score).

Risk Categories

- **Low risk (<10%):** lifestyle only.
- **Intermediate risk (10–19%):** lifestyle; consider statin if LDL-C ≥3.5, non-HDL ≥4.3, or ApoB ≥1.2.
- **High risk (≥20% or diabetes, CKD, clinical ASCVD):** statin therapy recommended.

Lifestyle Management (all patients)

- Heart-healthy diet (Mediterranean, DASH).

- Exercise: ≥150 min/week moderate-intensity.
- Weight management (BMI 18.5–24.9).
- Smoking cessation, limit alcohol.

Pharmacologic Therapy

- **First-line:** statins (atorvastatin, rosuvastatin).
- **Targets:**
    - ≥50% LDL-C reduction, OR
    - LDL-C <2.0 mmol/L (high risk).
- **Add-on therapy (if not at target):** ezetimibe, PCSK9 inhibitor (specialist).
- Monitor liver enzymes, CK only if symptoms.

Follow-Up

- Repeat lipids: 6–12 weeks after initiation or dose change.
- Annual lipid check once stable.
- Monitor adherence, side effects, ASCVD risk factors.

Referral

- **ED:** not typically indicated for dyslipidemia.
- **Specialist (lipid clinic/cardiology):**
    o Familial hypercholesterolemia (very high LDL-C).
    o Statin intolerance despite multiple trials.
    o High-risk patients not achieving targets on statin + ezetimibe.

Primary Care Management

- Most cases of elevated cholesterol and moderate ASCVD risk.
- Long-term monitoring and lifestyle counseling.
- Initiating and titrating statin therapy.

19. Angina & Acute Coronary Syndrome (ACS)

Definitions

- **Stable angina:** predictable, exertional chest pain, relieved by rest/nitro.
- **Unstable angina:** new, worsening, or occurring at rest; no biomarker rise.
- **NSTEMI/STEMI:** ACS with troponin elevation ± ST changes.

Risk Factors

- Hypertension, dyslipidemia, diabetes, smoking, family history, obesity, sedentary lifestyle.

Diagnosis in Office

- History: exertional chest pain, relieved by rest/nitro, radiation (jaw, arm), associated SOB, diaphoresis, nausea.
- Exam: may be normal; check vitals, murmurs, signs of HF.

- ECG: if available → look for ischemic changes (ST depression/elevation, T inversion).
- Labs (troponin) → not usually available in office; arrange ED.

Initial Office Management

- **Stable angina:**
    - Sublingual nitroglycerin PRN.
    - Long-term: ASA 81 mg daily, statin, consider beta-blocker/ACEi if comorbidities.
    - Risk factor modification.
- **ACS suspected (unstable angina, NSTEMI, STEMI):**
    - Give ASA 160–325 mg chewable immediately.
    - Nitro if SBP >90 and no contraindications.
    - Oxygen if SpO_2 <90%.
    - Call EMS → urgent ED transfer.

Referral

- **ED (urgent):** all ACS (unstable angina, NSTEMI, STEMI).
- **Cardiology (non-urgent):** stable angina not controlled with medical

therapy, abnormal stress test, recurrent angina, or planning revascularization.

Primary Care Management

- Confirmed stable angina with cardiology input.
- Ongoing risk factor management (HTN, diabetes, dyslipidemia, smoking cessation, weight).
- Long-term secondary prevention: ASA, statin, ACEi/ARB, beta-blocker as indicated.

Pocket Box – Office Angina/ACS Quick Reference

- **Step 1:** History + vitals + ECG if available.
- **Step 2:**
  - Stable angina → risk factor control, ASA, statin, PRN nitro.
  - Suspected ACS → ASA, nitro (if safe), O_2 (if hypoxic), EMS transfer.

Step 3: Refer cardiology for ongoing management.

20. Heart Failure (HFrEF & HFpEF)

Definitions

- **HFrEF:** LVEF ≤40% (systolic dysfunction).
- **HFpEF:** LVEF ≥50% (diastolic dysfunction).
- **HFmrEF:** mid-range EF 41–49% (treated similar to HFrEF).

Common Causes

- Ischemic heart disease (most common in Canada).
- Hypertension.
- Valvular heart disease.
- Arrhythmias.
- Cardiomyopathies (alcohol, viral, genetic).

Diagnosis (Office Level)

- Symptoms: dyspnea, orthopnea, PND, fatigue, edema, weight gain.

- Signs: JVP elevation, rales, S3 gallop, hepatomegaly, peripheral edema.
- Investigations (often arranged outpatient):
    - ECG (arrhythmia, ischemia, LVH).
    - CXR (pulmonary edema, cardiomegaly).
    - BNP/NT-proBNP (if available).
    - Echocardiogram → definitive (ordered via cardiology).
    - Labs: CBC, electrolytes, creatinine, TSH, LFTs.

Initial Office Management

- **All patients:**
    - Lifestyle: sodium restriction, daily weights, fluid balance, exercise as tolerated.
    - Vaccinations: influenza, pneumococcal.
- **HFrEF:**
    - ACEi/ARB/ARNI.
    - Beta-blocker (bisoprolol, metoprolol succinate, carvedilol).
    - MRA (spironolactone, eplerenone).
    - SGLT2 inhibitor (dapagliflozin, empagliflozin).

- o Diuretics (furosemide) for symptoms (not mortality benefit).
- **HFpEF:**
  - o Control BP, treat comorbidities (HTN, AF, diabetes).
  - o SGLT2 inhibitor may reduce hospitalizations.
  - o Diuretics for fluid overload.

Follow-Up

- Monitor weight, symptoms, BP, renal function, electrolytes.
- Adjust therapy stepwise.
- Reassess every 1–3 months when unstable; stable patients every 6–12 months.

Referral

- **ED (urgent):** acute decompensated HF (severe dyspnea, hypoxia, pulmonary edema, shock).
- **Specialist (non-urgent):**
  - o Cardiology for all new HF diagnoses.
  - o Refractory symptoms despite guideline-directed therapy.

- Suspected advanced HF (LVAD/transplant).

Primary Care Management

- Long-term monitoring of stable HF.
- Initiating/adjusting therapy per guidelines.
- Managing comorbidities (HTN, AF, diabetes).
- Palliative/supportive care discussions in advanced stages.

Pocket Box – Office Heart Failure Quick Reference

- **Step 1:** History (dyspnea, orthopnea, edema), exam (JVP, S3, rales).
- **Step 2:** ECG, labs, CXR; arrange echo.
- **Step 3:**
    - **HFrEF:** ACEi/ARB/ARNI + beta-blocker + MRA + SGLT2i; diuretics for symptoms.
    - **HFpEF:** control BP, treat comorbidities, SGLT2i, diuretics.
- **Step 4:**

- Acute decompensation → ED.

Stable → manage in office, refer cardiology.

21. Arrhythmias (AF, SVT, Bradyarrhythmias)

Common Arrhythmias in Primary Care

- **Atrial fibrillation (AF):** irregularly irregular rhythm, palpitations, stroke risk.
- **Supraventricular tachycardia (SVT):** sudden onset/offset, rapid palpitations.
- **Bradyarrhythmias:** sinus bradycardia, AV block.
- **Other:** PVCs, PACs (often benign).

Diagnosis in Office

- ECG: essential to confirm type of arrhythmia.
- History: palpitations, syncope, chest pain, SOB.
- Exam: pulse rate/rhythm, BP, heart sounds.
- Labs: electrolytes, thyroid function, CBC.
- Consider Holter monitor/event recorder for intermittent arrhythmia.

Initial Office Management

Atrial Fibrillation (AF)

- Assess stability (vitals, chest pain, syncope, shock).
- Rate control (beta-blocker, diltiazem) if symptomatic.
- Anticoagulation based on **CHA$_2$DS$_2$-VASc** score (warfarin or DOAC).
- Address reversible causes (thyroid, alcohol, infection, sleep apnea).

Supraventricular Tachycardia (SVT)

- Stable: vagal maneuvers (Valsalva, carotid massage).
- If unsuccessful and persistent → refer ED for adenosine/cardioversion.
- Recurrent → cardiology for ablation consideration.

Bradyarrhythmias

- Stable sinus bradycardia often benign (athletes, sleep).
- Symptomatic (syncope, dizziness, hypotension): urgent ED referral.
- Check medications (beta-blockers, digoxin, CCBs).

Referral

- **ED (urgent):**
  - Hemodynamic instability with tachy- or bradyarrhythmia.
  - New-onset AF with chest pain, HF, hypotension.
  - Symptomatic bradycardia or high-grade AV block.
- **Specialist (cardiology, non-urgent):**
  - New AF for anticoagulation/long-term rhythm strategy.
  - Recurrent SVT.
  - Symptomatic or unexplained bradycardia requiring pacemaker consideration.

Primary Care Management

- Stable, asymptomatic AF with cardiology input (anticoagulation, rate control).
- Benign ectopy (PACs, PVCs) with reassurance.
- Long-term monitoring of patients post-cardiology assessment.

Pocket Box – Office Arrhythmia Quick Reference

- **Step 1:** ECG on all suspected arrhythmias.
- **Step 2:** Labs → electrolytes, TSH, CBC.
- **Step 3:**
    - **AF:** rate control, anticoagulate, refer cardiology.
    - **SVT:** vagal maneuvers → if fails, ED.
    - **Brady:** if symptomatic, ED; if asymptomatic, review meds + monitor.

Step 4: Ongoing primary care role in risk factor control + monitoring.

22. Stroke & Transient Ischemic Attack (TIA)

Definitions

- **Stroke:** acute neurological deficit >24h, due to ischemia or hemorrhage.
- **TIA:** focal neurological deficit <24h, usually <1h, without infarction.

Risk Factors

- Hypertension (strongest modifiable).
- Atrial fibrillation.
- Diabetes, dyslipidemia, smoking, obesity.
- Prior stroke/TIA.

Diagnosis in Office

- Symptoms: sudden onset weakness, numbness, facial droop, speech difficulty, vision loss, imbalance.
- Screen: FAST (Face, Arm, Speech, Time).
- Exam: neuro deficits (motor, sensory, speech, vision, gait).

- BP measurement.
- ECG (AF).
- Labs: glucose (exclude hypoglycemia mimicking stroke).

Initial Office Management

- **If stroke suspected:**
  - Call EMS immediately → "Stroke Code" to ED.
  - Do NOT delay with office imaging or labs.
  - Note symptom onset time (eligibility for thrombolysis/thrombectomy).
- **If TIA suspected (symptoms resolved):**
  - ASA 160–325 mg immediately.
  - Urgent referral to ED/stroke clinic for imaging and secondary prevention.

Referral

- **ED (urgent):**
  - All suspected strokes.
  - All TIAs within past 48h (high early stroke risk).
- **Specialist (non-urgent):**

- Stroke clinic follow-up for secondary prevention (antiplatelets, statins, anticoagulation if AF, BP control).

Primary Care Management

- Long-term secondary prevention:
  - Antiplatelet (ASA, clopidogrel, or ASA/dipyridamole).
  - Statin (high-intensity).
  - Anticoagulation for AF.
  - BP control (<130/80 in most).
  - Lifestyle modification (smoking cessation, diet, exercise, weight management).
- Monitor mood and cognition post-stroke (depression, dementia common).
- Rehab coordination (physio, OT, speech therapy).

Pocket Box – Office Stroke/TIA Quick Reference

- **Step 1:** Recognize symptoms (FAST).
- **Step 2:**
  - Stroke → EMS immediately, document onset.

- TIA → ASA now, urgent ED/stroke clinic referral.

Step 3: Long-term secondary prevention (antiplatelet, statin, anticoagulation if AF, BP/lifestyle control).

This page has been left intentionally blank

Section 2: Respiratory Medicine

23. Asthma

Diagnosis

- Symptoms: wheeze, SOB, chest tightness, cough (often worse at night/early morning).
- Variable, reversible airflow obstruction.
- Spirometry: FEV_1/FVC <0.75–0.80 + improvement post-bronchodilator.
- Consider peak flow variability if spirometry not available.

Triggers

- Allergens (dust, pollen, pets).
- Viral infections.
- Exercise, cold air.
- Irritants (smoke, pollution).
- Medications (NSAIDs, beta-blockers).

Initial Office Management

- **Mild asthma (infrequent):** as-needed low-dose ICS-formoterol (preferred) OR SABA + ICS.

- **Persistent asthma:** daily low-dose ICS ± as-needed ICS-formoterol.
- **Moderate-severe:** stepwise add LABA, LTRA, higher ICS dose, biologics (specialist).
- Provide asthma action plan.
- Vaccinations: influenza, pneumococcal.

Acute Exacerbation (in office)

- Assess severity: vitals, O_2 sat, ability to speak, accessory muscle use.
- O_2 if SpO_2 <90%.
- Salbutamol via MDI/spacer or neb q20min × 3.
- Add ipratropium if moderate-severe.
- Oral prednisone 40–50 mg × 5–7 days if moderate-severe.
- **Refer to ED if:** poor response, hypoxia, severe distress, altered LOC.

Follow-Up

- Review control every 3 months.
- Spirometry q1–2 years.
- Step up if uncontrolled, step down if controlled ≥3 months.

Referral

- **ED (urgent):** severe exacerbation (silent chest, hypoxia, altered LOC).
- **Specialist (respirology, non-urgent):**
    - Severe asthma uncontrolled on high-dose ICS/LABA.
    - Frequent exacerbations.
    - Unclear diagnosis.

Primary Care Management

- Most mild-moderate asthma.
- Initiation and titration of ICS/LABA.
- Monitoring, education, inhaler technique, action plan.

Pocket Box – Office Asthma Quick Reference

- **Step 1:** Confirm diagnosis with spirometry.
- **Step 2:** Start ICS (low-dose daily or as-needed ICS-formoterol).
- **Step 3:** Provide action plan, check inhaler technique.
- **Step 4:** Exacerbation → O_2, salbutamol ± ipratropium, prednisone, refer if severe.

Step 5: Refer respirology if uncontrolled/severe.

24. Chronic Obstructive Pulmonary Disease (COPD)

Diagnosis

- Symptoms: chronic cough, sputum, dyspnea, recurrent infections.
- Risk factors: smoking (primary), occupational exposures, biomass fuels.
- Spirometry: FEV_1/FVC <0.70 post-bronchodilator (not fully reversible).
- Consider alpha-1 antitrypsin deficiency if <45 years or non-smoker.

Severity (GOLD Classification by FEV_1 % predicted)

- Mild: ≥80%
- Moderate: 50–79%
- Severe: 30–49%
- Very severe: <30%

Initial Office Management

- **All patients:**

- Smoking cessation (most important).
- Vaccinations: influenza, pneumococcal, COVID.
- Pulmonary rehab, exercise.
- **Pharmacotherapy (stepwise):**
  - Mild symptoms: short-acting bronchodilator (SABA or SAMA).
  - Persistent: LABA or LAMA.
  - Severe or frequent exacerbations: LABA + LAMA ± ICS (triple therapy).
  - ICS reserved for eosinophilic phenotype or frequent exacerbations.
- Oxygen therapy if chronic hypoxemia (PaO_2 ≤55 mmHg or SpO_2 ≤88%).

Exacerbation (in office)

- Symptoms: worsening dyspnea, cough, sputum volume/purulence.
- O_2 if SpO_2 <90%.
- Salbutamol ± ipratropium (MDI/nebulizer).
- Oral prednisone 40 mg × 5 days.
- Antibiotics if ↑sputum purulence + volume + dyspnea (e.g., amoxicillin-clavulanate, doxycycline).

- **Refer ED if:** severe hypoxemia, respiratory distress, altered LOC, hemodynamic instability.

Follow-Up

- Spirometry q1–2 years.
- Reassess inhaler technique and adherence every visit.
- Monitor for comorbidities: CVD, osteoporosis, depression.

Referral

- **ED (urgent):** severe exacerbation, hypoxemia, altered mental status.
- **Specialist (respirology, non-urgent):**
    - Uncertain diagnosis.
    - Frequent exacerbations or hospitalizations.
    - Severe COPD for advanced therapies (oxygen, lung transplant).

Primary Care Management

- Stable mild-moderate COPD.
- Smoking cessation counseling.

- Initiating and titrating inhaled therapies.
- Routine vaccinations, comorbidity management.

Pocket Box – Office COPD Quick Reference

- **Step 1:** Confirm with spirometry (post-BD FEV_1/FVC <0.70).
- **Step 2:** Lifestyle: smoking cessation, vaccines, rehab.
- **Step 3:** Inhaler: SABA/SAMA → LABA/LAMA → triple therapy if severe.
- **Step 4:** Exacerbation → O_2, salbutamol/ipratropium, prednisone, ± antibiotics.
- **Step 5:** Refer ED if unstable; respirology if severe or frequent exacerbations.

25. Pneumonia

Diagnosis

- Symptoms: fever, cough, sputum, pleuritic chest pain, dyspnea.
- Exam: crackles, bronchial breath sounds, dullness to percussion.
- CXR: consolidation (required for diagnosis if available).
- Labs (if arranged): CBC (↑WBC), CRP.

Common Causes

- **Community-acquired (CAP):** *Streptococcus pneumoniae* (most common), *H. influenzae*, atypicals (Mycoplasma, Chlamydophila).
- **Viral:** influenza, RSV, COVID-19.
- **Hospital-acquired:** gram-negative bacilli, *Staph aureus*.
- **Special:** aspiration pneumonia (anaerobes).

Severity Assessment (decides site of care)

- **CURB-65:** Confusion, Urea >7, RR ≥30, BP <90/60, Age ≥65.
    - 0–1 → outpatient.
    - 2 → consider admission.
    - 3–5 → hospital/ICU.

Initial Office Management

- **Outpatient, otherwise healthy:** amoxicillin OR doxycycline OR macrolide.
- **Comorbidities:** amoxicillin-clavulanate + macrolide OR respiratory fluoroquinolone.
- **Supportive:** rest, fluids, antipyretics, O_2 if hypoxic.
- **Avoid empiric antibiotics** in viral pneumonia (COVID, influenza).

When to Refer to ED (Urgent)

- Hypoxemia (SpO_2 <90%).
- Respiratory distress, tachypnea >30.
- Hypotension, sepsis.
- Confusion, altered mental status.
- CURB-65 ≥2.

When to Refer to Specialists (Non-Urgent)

- Recurrent pneumonia → respirology work-up (bronchiectasis, immunodeficiency).
- Non-resolving pneumonia (rule out malignancy, TB).
- Severe or unusual pathogens (ID specialist).

Primary Care Management

- Mild outpatient CAP (stable, CURB-65 0–1).
- Viral pneumonia without hypoxia (supportive care).
- Monitoring response (should improve in 48–72h).
- Vaccinations: pneumococcal, influenza, COVID boosters.

Pocket Box – Office Pneumonia Quick Reference

- **Step 1:** Suspect with fever, cough, chest pain, dyspnea → confirm with CXR if possible.
- **Step 2:** Assess severity with CURB-65.
- **Step 3:**

- Stable, low risk → outpatient oral antibiotics.
- High risk/unstable → ED referral.

Step 4: Follow up 48–72h; refer if no improvement.

26. Tuberculosis (TB)

Epidemiology

- Higher risk in: Indigenous populations, immigrants from endemic regions, immunocompromised (HIV, transplant), homeless, IV drug use.
- Public health–notifiable disease in Canada.

Types

- **Latent TB Infection (LTBI):** positive TST/IGRA, no symptoms, normal CXR.
- **Active TB (pulmonary):** cough >2–3 weeks, hemoptysis, fever, night sweats, weight loss, abnormal CXR.
- **Extrapulmonary TB:** lymph nodes, bone, CNS, genitourinary.

Diagnosis in Office

- Suspicion: chronic cough, weight loss, fever, night sweats, hemoptysis.

- Risk assessment (travel, contacts, immunocompromise).
- Investigations (arranged via public health/hospital):
  - Tuberculin skin test (TST) or IGRA (latent TB).
  - CXR (upper lobe infiltrates, cavitations).
  - Sputum AFB smear/culture + NAAT (definitive for active TB).

Initial Office Management

- If **suspected active TB:**
  - Mask patient, isolate, avoid waiting room exposure.
  - Do NOT start treatment in office → urgent referral to public health/infectious disease.
- If **latent TB:**
  - Refer to public health/ID for therapy (isoniazid, rifampin regimens).

When to Refer to ED (Urgent)

- Severe respiratory distress or hemoptysis.

- Very ill, unstable, or highly infectious patient.
- CNS TB suspicion (meningitis).

When to Refer to Specialists (Non-Urgent)

- **Infectious Diseases/Public Health:** ALL confirmed or suspected TB (latent or active).
- **Respirology:** complicated pulmonary TB, structural lung disease.
- **Other specialties:** extrapulmonary TB (neuro, ortho, GU).

Primary Care Management

- Screening high-risk populations with TST/IGRA.
- Coordinating with public health for latent TB therapy.
- Monitoring medication adherence and side effects (hepatotoxicity).
- Supporting vaccination and general health.

Pocket Box – Office TB Quick Reference

- **Step 1:** Suspect TB if chronic cough, weight loss, fever, night sweats, hemoptysis.
- **Step 2:** Order CXR, TST/IGRA; sputum AFB if suspected active.
- **Step 3:**
    - Active TB → isolate, mask, urgent referral to ID/public health.
    - Latent TB → refer for preventive therapy.

Step 4: PCP role → screening, follow-up, adherence support.

27. Pulmonary Embolism (PE)

Risk Factors

- Recent surgery/immobilization
- Cancer
- Pregnancy, postpartum, OCP/HRT use
- Prior DVT/PE
- Obesity, thrombophilia (inherited/acquired)

Clinical Presentation

- Dyspnea, pleuritic chest pain, cough, hemoptysis
- Tachycardia, tachypnea, hypoxemia
- Syncope (massive PE)
- Signs of DVT (swollen, tender calf)

Diagnosis in Office

- Assess clinical probability (e.g., **Wells score**):
  - Low → order D-dimer.
  - High → skip D-dimer, send for imaging.

- Definitive imaging: CTPA (gold standard), V/Q scan if contraindication.
- D-dimer useful only in low-intermediate risk patients.

Initial Office Management

- If PE suspected:
    - Oxygen if hypoxemic.
    - Avoid delay → arrange urgent ED transfer.
    - Do NOT start anticoagulation in office unless long delay expected AND high clinical suspicion.

When to Refer to ED (Urgent)

- All suspected PE (requires imaging and urgent treatment).
- Hemodynamic instability → "massive PE" (shock, hypotension).

When to Refer to Specialists (Non-Urgent)

- **Hematology:** recurrent PE, thrombophilia work-up, anticoagulation management.
- **Oncology:** cancer-associated thrombosis.
- **Cardiology/Respirology:** chronic thromboembolic pulmonary hypertension.

Primary Care Management

- Long-term anticoagulation monitoring (warfarin INR checks, DOAC adherence).
- Managing comorbidities and risk reduction (weight, smoking cessation, mobility).
- Supporting transitions after specialist/ED care.

Pocket Box – Office PE Quick Reference

- **Step 1:** Suspect PE with dyspnea, pleuritic chest pain, tachycardia, DVT signs.
- **Step 2:** Calculate Wells score.
    - Low → D-dimer.
    - High → direct imaging/referral.
- **Step 3:**
    - Oxygen if hypoxic.

- EMS transfer to ED for definitive imaging and anticoagulation.

Step 4: PCP role = long-term anticoagulation follow-up, prevention.

28. Obstructive Sleep Apnea (OSA)

Risk Factors

- Obesity (BMI >30)
- Male sex, age >40
- Large neck circumference (>40 cm)
- Craniofacial abnormalities (retrognathia)
- Family history
- Alcohol, sedatives

Clinical Presentation

- Loud snoring, witnessed apneas
- Daytime sleepiness, fatigue
- Morning headaches
- Poor concentration, mood changes
- Hypertension, resistant HTN
- Nocturia

Diagnosis in Office

- **Screening tools:** STOP-BANG, Epworth Sleepiness Scale.

- Physical exam: BMI, neck circumference, nasal obstruction.
- Definitive: polysomnography (sleep study).

Initial Office Management

- Lifestyle: weight loss, exercise, avoid alcohol/sedatives, positional therapy.
- Manage comorbidities (HTN, diabetes, AF).
- Educate about driving risk (daytime sleepiness = ↑ accident risk).
- Arrange sleep study referral for confirmation.

Treatment (Specialist Initiated, PCP Support)

- CPAP (first-line for moderate-severe OSA).
- Oral appliances (mild-moderate, CPAP intolerant).
- Surgery (ENT for selected cases).

When to Refer to ED (Urgent)

- Rarely ED unless severe hypoxemia or overlap with acute illness.

When to Refer to Specialists (Non-Urgent)

- **Sleep medicine / Respirology:** suspected OSA for diagnostic testing + CPAP initiation.
- **ENT / Dental Sleep Specialist:** structural issues, oral appliances.

Primary Care Management

- Screening high-risk patients.
- Lifestyle counselling.
- Coordinating referrals for sleep study and CPAP initiation.
- Long-term follow-up of adherence, comorbidity management.

Pocket Box – Office OSA Quick Reference

- **Step 1:** Screen with STOP-BANG/Epworth in at-risk patients.
- **Step 2:** Lifestyle advice (weight loss, avoid alcohol/sedatives).

- **Step 3:** Refer for polysomnography.

Step 4: Support CPAP adherence, monitor comorbidities.

This page has been left intentionally blank

Section 3: Endocrinology & Metabolism

29. Diabetes Mellitus

Diagnosis *(need 2 abnormal tests unless symptomatic with random glucose)*

- FPG ≥7.0 mmol/L.
- A1C ≥6.5% (not for diagnosis in children, pregnancy, suspected type 1).
- 2-hr PG in 75g OGTT ≥11.1 mmol/L.
- Random PG ≥11.1 mmol/L + symptoms.

Types

- **Type 1 DM:** autoimmune beta-cell destruction, insulin dependent.
- **Type 2 DM:** insulin resistance + relative deficiency, most common.
- **Gestational DM:** glucose intolerance first recognized in pregnancy.
- **Secondary causes:** steroids, pancreatic disease, endocrinopathies.

Initial Office Assessment

- Confirm diagnosis with repeat test (if asymptomatic).

- Baseline labs: A1C, FPG, lipid profile, creatinine/eGFR, electrolytes, urine ACR, LFTs, TSH (if type 1).
- Physical exam: BMI, waist circumference, BP, foot exam (sensation, pulses, skin).
- Screen for complications: retinopathy (ophthalmology), neuropathy, nephropathy.

Initial Management

- **Lifestyle (all patients):**
  - Diet: balanced, Mediterranean/DASH style.
  - Weight reduction if overweight.
  - Exercise: ≥150 min/week aerobic + resistance.
  - Smoking cessation.
- **Pharmacologic (T2DM):**
  - First-line: **Metformin** (if no contraindications).
  - Add based on comorbidities:
    - ASCVD: SGLT2 inhibitor or GLP-1 agonist.
    - HF or CKD: SGLT2 inhibitor preferred.
  - Individualize A1C target (≤7% for most).
- **T1DM:** Insulin therapy (basal-bolus or pump).

Follow-Up

- A1C q3 months until stable, then q6 months.
- BP target: <130/80 if high CV risk.
- Annual screening: lipids, kidney (ACR), eye exam, foot exam.
- Vaccinations: influenza, pneumococcal, hepatitis B if at risk.

Referral

- **ED (urgent):** suspected DKA or HHS (polyuria, polydipsia, vomiting, confusion, Kussmaul breathing).
- **Specialist (endocrinology, non-urgent):**
    - Type 1 DM (initial + ongoing care).
    - Uncontrolled T2DM despite multiple agents/insulin.
    - Unclear diagnosis or atypical diabetes.
    - Pregnancy (gestational or pre-existing DM).

Primary Care Management

- Most stable T2DM patients.

- Initiate and adjust oral/GLP-1/SGLT2 therapy.
- Lifestyle coaching and complication screening.
- Long-term monitoring and prevention of CVD.

Pocket Box – Office Diabetes Quick Reference

- **Step 1:** Diagnose with FPG, A1C, or OGTT (confirm if needed).
- **Step 2:** Baseline labs + complication screen.
- **Step 3:** Lifestyle changes for all; start Metformin if T2DM.
- **Step 4:** Add SGLT2i/GLP-1 if ASCVD/CKD/HF.
- **Step 5:** A1C q3–6 months, annual eyes/feet/kidneys.

Step 6: Refer endo for T1DM, pregnancy, or refractory T2DM.

30. Thyroid Disease

Hypothyroidism

- **Causes:** Hashimoto's thyroiditis (most common), post-radioiodine/surgery, medications (amiodarone, lithium).
- **Symptoms:** fatigue, weight gain, cold intolerance, constipation, dry skin, depression.
- **Diagnosis:** ↑TSH + ↓Free T4 (overt); ↑TSH + normal T4 (subclinical).
- **Treatment:** Levothyroxine (dose based on weight/age, adjust q6–8 weeks).
- **Referral:** endo if pregnancy, children, refractory, pituitary disease.

Hyperthyroidism

- **Causes:** Graves' disease, toxic multinodular goiter, thyroiditis, medications (amiodarone).
- **Symptoms:** weight loss, heat intolerance, palpitations, tremor, anxiety, diarrhea.
- **Diagnosis:** ↓TSH + ↑Free T4/T3.
- **Initial management:**
    - Beta-blocker (symptom control).

- o Antithyroid drugs (methimazole, PTU if pregnancy/first trimester).
- o Radioiodine or surgery (definitive, specialist-based).
- **Referral:** all suspected hyperthyroidism to endocrinology.

Thyroid Nodules

- **Presentation:** palpable neck lump, incidental on imaging.
- **Assessment:**
  - o TSH first.
  - o Ultrasound to assess nodule characteristics.
  - o Fine needle aspiration (FNA) if suspicious features or >1 cm (per guidelines).
- **Referral:** endocrinology/ENT for suspicious or indeterminate nodules.

When to Refer to ED (Urgent)

- Thyroid storm (fever, tachycardia, confusion, arrhythmia).
- Myxedema coma (hypothermia, bradycardia, altered mental status).

Primary Care Management

- Most hypothyroidism cases (stable on levothyroxine).
- Monitoring TSH q6–12 months.
- Long-term follow-up for subclinical hypothyroidism if not treated.
- Early recognition and referral of hyperthyroidism/nodules.

Pocket Box – Office Thyroid Quick Reference

- **Step 1:** TSH as initial test.
- **Step 2:**
  - ↑TSH + ↓T4 → hypothyroid → levothyroxine.
  - ↓TSH + ↑T4/T3 → hyperthyroid → beta-blocker + refer.
  - Nodule → TSH + ultrasound ± FNA.

Step 3: Refer urgently if thyroid storm or myxedema coma.

31. Adrenal & Pituitary Disorders

Adrenal Disorders

Adrenal Insufficiency (Addison's Disease, Secondary AI)

- **Causes:** autoimmune (primary), pituitary disease (secondary), chronic steroids (suppression).
- **Symptoms:** fatigue, weight loss, hyperpigmentation (primary), hypotension, hyponatremia, hyperkalemia.
- **Diagnosis:** low AM cortisol + ACTH stimulation test.
- **Treatment:** hydrocortisone ± fludrocortisone (primary AI).
- **ED referral:** adrenal crisis (shock, vomiting, confusion → urgent IV hydrocortisone + fluids).

Cushing's Syndrome

- **Causes:** chronic steroid use (most common), pituitary adenoma (Cushing's disease), adrenal tumour, ectopic ACTH.

- **Symptoms:** central obesity, striae, moon face, proximal weakness, HTN, diabetes, mood changes.
- **Diagnosis:** low-dose dex suppression test, 24h urine cortisol, late-night salivary cortisol.
- **Referral:** endocrinology for all suspected cases.

Pheochromocytoma

- **Symptoms:** paroxysmal HTN, headaches, palpitations, sweating.
- **Diagnosis:** plasma or urine metanephrines.
- **Referral:** endocrinology + surgery.

Pituitary Disorders

Hypopituitarism

- Causes: pituitary adenoma, surgery, radiation, infarction (Sheehan's).
- Symptoms: fatigue, low libido, amenorrhea, hypothyroidism, adrenal insufficiency.
- Diagnosis: low pituitary + target hormones.
- Referral: endocrinology.

Pituitary Adenomas

- Prolactinoma (most common): galactorrhea, amenorrhea, infertility, low libido.
- Acromegaly (GH excess): enlarged hands/feet, coarse features, diabetes.
- Cushing's disease (ACTH-secreting).
- Non-functioning adenomas: mass effect (headache, visual field loss).
- Diagnosis: MRI pituitary + hormonal assays.
- Treatment: medical (e.g., dopamine agonists for prolactinoma) or surgery (neurosurgery).

When to Refer to ED (Urgent)

- Adrenal crisis (shock, severe dehydration, confusion).
- Pituitary apoplexy (sudden headache, vision loss, ophthalmoplegia).
- Hypertensive crisis with pheochromocytoma.

Primary Care Management

- Long-term hydrocortisone replacement for Addison's (shared care with endocrinology).
- Monitoring prolactinomas on dopamine agonists (endo-guided).

- Identifying and referring suspected pituitary/adrenal disorders.

Pocket Box – Office Adrenal & Pituitary Quick Reference

- **Step 1:** Suspect adrenal insufficiency → AM cortisol, urgent ED if crisis.
- **Step 2:** Cushing's features → screen (low-dose dex test) → refer endo.
- **Step 3:** Paroxysmal HTN/headaches → plasma metanephrines → refer endo.

Step 4: Pituitary mass symptoms (amenorrhea, galactorrhea, visual changes) → MRI → endocrinology/neurosurgery.

32. Osteoporosis & Bone Health

Definition

- Low bone mass + microarchitectural deterioration → ↑ fracture risk.
- Diagnosed by bone mineral density (BMD) via DXA scan.

Risk Factors

- Age >65, postmenopausal women.
- Family history of hip fracture.
- Low body weight (BMI <20).
- Smoking, alcohol excess.
- Glucocorticoid use (>3 months).
- Chronic diseases: RA, CKD, malabsorption, hypogonadism.

Diagnosis & Screening

- **Screening (per Osteoporosis Canada):**
    - Women ≥65 and men ≥65.
    - Postmenopausal women and men 50–64 with risk factors.

- **Tests:**
  - DXA scan (lumbar spine, hip).
  - FRAX or CAROC tool to calculate fracture risk.
  - Labs: Ca, phosphate, creatinine, vitamin D, ALP, TSH (secondary causes).

Initial Office Management

- Lifestyle: weight-bearing/resistance exercise, smoking cessation, reduce alcohol.
- Calcium intake 1200 mg/day (diet preferred).
- Vitamin D 800–2000 IU/day.
- Fall prevention strategies.

Pharmacologic Therapy (if high fracture risk)

- First-line: oral bisphosphonates (alendronate, risedronate).
- Alternatives: denosumab, raloxifene, HRT (women), teriparatide (severe).
- Treatment duration: bisphosphonates typically 3–5 years, then reassess.

Follow-Up

- Monitor adherence, side effects (GI with bisphosphonates, ONJ rare).
- Repeat BMD every 2–3 years.
- Reassess fracture risk periodically.

When to Refer to ED (Urgent)

- Acute fragility fracture (hip, vertebral).
- Symptomatic hypercalcemia.

When to Refer to Specialists (Non-Urgent)

- Endocrinology/rheumatology: severe or refractory osteoporosis, multiple fragility fractures, secondary causes.
- Orthopedics: fracture management.

Primary Care Management

- Screening and diagnosis of osteoporosis.
- Lifestyle counseling and vitamin D/calcium supplementation.

- Initiating and monitoring bisphosphonate therapy in straightforward cases.

> **Pocket Box – Office Osteoporosis Quick Reference**
>
> - **Step 1:** Screen with DXA in women/men ≥65 or earlier with risks.
> - **Step 2:** Labs to rule out secondary causes.
> - **Step 3:** Lifestyle + Vit D + Ca for all.
> - **Step 4:** Bisphosphonate if high risk or fragility fracture.
>
> **Step 5:** Repeat DXA 2–3 years; refer endo if severe or refractory.

33. Obesity Management

Definition

- Chronic, relapsing disease characterized by excess body fat with health impact.
- **BMI ≥30** (adults) or **BMI ≥25** (Asian populations).
- Waist circumference >102 cm (men), >88 cm (women) = ↑ cardiometabolic risk.

Contributing Factors

- Genetics, environment, diet, physical inactivity.
- Medications (antipsychotics, antidepressants, steroids, insulin).
- Endocrine disorders (hypothyroidism, Cushing's, PCOS).
- Psychosocial factors.

Complications

- Type 2 diabetes, HTN, dyslipidemia, ASCVD.

- OSA, GERD, NAFLD.
- Osteoarthritis.
- Depression, stigma, reduced quality of life.

Initial Office Management

- **Approach:** empathetic, non-judgmental, chronic disease model.
- **Lifestyle:**
    - Diet: caloric restriction, Mediterranean/DASH-style eating.
    - Physical activity: 150 min/week aerobic + resistance training.
    - Behavioural therapy/support groups.
- **Pharmacologic options (if BMI ≥30 or ≥27 with comorbidities):**
    - Orlistat.
    - GLP-1 agonists (liraglutide, semaglutide).
    - Naltrexone-bupropion.
- **Surgical options:**
    - Bariatric surgery if BMI ≥40 OR ≥35 with comorbidities, after failed conservative therapy.

Follow-Up

- Regular weight, BMI, waist circumference.
- Monitor for complications: diabetes, HTN, OSA, NAFLD.
- Medication side effects (GI with orlistat, nausea with GLP-1).

When to Refer to ED (Urgent)

- Rarely ED unless acute complication (e.g., SBO post-bariatric surgery).

When to Refer to Specialists (Non-Urgent)

- Bariatric medicine or surgery program.
- Dietitian, psychologist/psychiatry.
- Endocrinology if complex comorbidities.

Primary Care Management

- Screening, diagnosis, and monitoring.
- Lifestyle counselling and initiation of pharmacotherapy.
- Long-term follow-up and support.
- Coordination with allied health and specialists.

Pocket Box – Office Obesity Quick Reference

- **Step 1:** Measure BMI + waist circumference.
- **Step 2:** Screen for comorbidities (DM, HTN, OSA, NAFLD).
- **Step 3:** Lifestyle: diet, exercise, behavioural.
- **Step 4:** Medications if BMI ≥30 or ≥27 + comorbidities.

Step 5: Refer bariatric surgery if BMI ≥40 or ≥35 + comorbidities.

34. Vitamin D Deficiency

Definition & Role

- Vitamin D = essential for calcium absorption & bone health.
- Deficiency → rickets (children), osteomalacia & osteoporosis (adults).

Risk Factors

- Limited sun exposure (northern latitudes, winter).
- Darker skin pigmentation.
- Elderly, institutionalized.
- Malabsorption (celiac, IBD, gastric bypass).
- Chronic kidney or liver disease.
- Medications: anticonvulsants, glucocorticoids.

Diagnosis

- Serum **25(OH)D level**:
    - Deficiency: <30 nmol/L.
    - Insufficient: 30–50 nmol/L.

- o   Adequate: >50 nmol/L (most adults).
- May see hypocalcemia, ↑PTH in severe deficiency.

Initial Office Management

- **Lifestyle:** safe sun exposure, diet (fortified milk, fatty fish, egg yolks).
- **Supplementation (adults):**
  - o   Routine: 800–2000 IU/day.
  - o   Deficiency: higher dose (e.g., 50,000 IU weekly × 6–8 weeks, then maintenance).
- **Children:** 400 IU/day (infants), 600–1000 IU/day (older kids if risk).

Follow-Up

- Recheck 25(OH)D after 3–4 months of therapy.
- Monitor calcium and renal function if high-dose supplementation.
- Long-term maintenance usually needed in at-risk groups.

When to Refer to ED (Urgent)

- Symptomatic hypocalcemia (tetany, seizures, arrhythmia).

When to Refer to Specialists (Non-Urgent)

- Endocrinology: refractory or unexplained deficiency, suspected metabolic bone disease, CKD-related bone-mineral disorder.
- Gastroenterology: malabsorption syndromes.

Primary Care Management

- Screening at-risk groups.
- Initiating and monitoring supplementation.
- Counselling on diet, lifestyle, and safe sun exposure.
- Managing most uncomplicated deficiency cases.

Pocket Box – Office Vitamin D Deficiency Quick Reference

- **Step 1:** Order 25(OH)D in at-risk patients.
- **Step 2:** <30 nmol/L = deficient → high-dose replacement.
- **Step 3:** Maintenance: 800–2000 IU/day in adults.

- **Step 4:** Recheck in 3–4 months; continue long-term in high-risk groups.

Step 5: Refer endo if refractory, severe, or metabolic bone disease suspected.

Section 4:
Gastroenterology

35. GERD, Dyspepsia & Peptic Ulcer Disease (PUD)

GERD (Gastroesophageal Reflux Disease)

- **Symptoms:** heartburn, regurgitation, chest discomfort, chronic cough/throat symptoms.
- **Red flags (need endoscopy):** dysphagia, odynophagia, weight loss, anemia, GI bleed, age >50 with new symptoms.
- **Diagnosis:** usually clinical; EGD if red flags or refractory.
- **Management:**
    - Lifestyle: weight loss, elevate head of bed, avoid late meals, reduce caffeine/alcohol, avoid trigger foods.
    - Pharmacologic: trial of PPI (omeprazole, pantoprazole) for 8 weeks.
    - H2 blockers if mild.
    - Long-term PPI for severe or erosive disease.
    - Surgery (fundoplication) in refractory cases.

Dyspepsia

- **Definition:** upper abdominal pain/discomfort, bloating, nausea.
- **Red flags (EGD needed):** weight loss, anemia, vomiting, GI bleed, progressive dysphagia, FHx GI cancer.
- **Diagnosis:**
    - Age <60 without red flags → test & treat *H. pylori*.
    - Age ≥60 or red flags → EGD.
- **Management:**
    - H. pylori positive → eradication (PPI + clarithromycin + amoxicillin/ metronidazole × 14 days).
    - Negative → PPI trial.

Peptic Ulcer Disease (PUD)

- **Causes:** H. pylori, NSAIDs, steroids, stress (critically ill).
- **Symptoms:** epigastric pain, dyspepsia, relief with food (duodenal), worse with food (gastric).
- **Diagnosis:** endoscopy = gold standard; H. pylori testing.
- **Management:**
    - Stop NSAIDs.
    - Eradicate H. pylori if positive.
    - PPI × 8 weeks.

- Surgery if complications (bleeding, perforation, obstruction).

When to Refer to ED (Urgent)

- GI bleeding (hematemesis, melena, hematochezia).
- Perforation (sudden severe abdominal pain, rigid abdomen).
- Severe dysphagia or obstruction.

When to Refer to Specialists (Non-Urgent)

- GI for endoscopy if red flags, refractory GERD, persistent dyspepsia.
- Complicated PUD (bleeding, stricture, recurrent).

Primary Care Management

- Most uncomplicated GERD and dyspepsia.
- Initial H. pylori testing & eradication.
- Short-term PPI use and lifestyle advice.
- Monitoring and reassessment.

Pocket Box – Office GERD/Dyspepsia/PUD Quick Reference

- **Step 1:** GERD suspected → trial PPI + lifestyle.
- **Step 2:** Dyspepsia → <60 test/treat H. pylori; ≥60 or red flags → EGD.
- **Step 3:** PUD → treat cause (H. pylori/NSAIDs) + PPI.

Step 4: Refer ED if bleeding, perforation, obstruction.

36. Irritable Bowel Syndrome (IBS) vs Inflammatory Bowel Disease (IBD)

IBS (Functional Disorder)

- **Symptoms:** recurrent abdominal pain + change in stool frequency/form, relieved by defecation.
- **Rome IV criteria:** symptoms ≥1 day/week in last 3 months, with ≥2 of: related to defecation, change in stool frequency, change in stool form.
- **Subtypes:** IBS-D (diarrhea), IBS-C (constipation), IBS-M (mixed).
- **Red flags (exclude IBD/cancer):** weight loss, anemia, nocturnal symptoms, blood in stool, onset >50.
- **Investigations (to exclude organic disease):** CBC, CRP or fecal calprotectin, celiac serology.

Management (IBS):

- Lifestyle/diet: low FODMAP diet, fiber (psyllium), hydration, stress reduction.
- Pharmacologic:
    - IBS-D: loperamide, bile acid binders.

- IBS-C: PEG, lubiprostone, linaclotide.
  - Antispasmodics (dicyclomine), low-dose TCA for pain.
- Psychological: CBT, mindfulness, reassurance.

IBD (Crohn's & Ulcerative Colitis)

- **Crohn's:** mouth to anus, skip lesions, transmural, fistulas.
- **UC:** continuous from rectum, mucosal only.
- **Symptoms:** chronic diarrhea, blood/mucus in stool, abdominal pain, weight loss, fatigue.
- **Extra-intestinal manifestations:** arthritis, uveitis, erythema nodosum, PSC.
- **Investigations:** CBC (anemia), CRP, ESR, stool cultures, fecal calprotectin. Definitive = colonoscopy with biopsy.

Management (IBD):

- Refer to gastroenterology for diagnosis & long-term management.
- PCP role: supportive care, vaccinations, mental health, monitoring.
- Acute flares: systemic steroids (specialist directed).

- Maintenance: 5-ASA, immunosuppressants, biologics (specialist).

When to Refer to ED (Urgent)

- Severe GI bleed.
- Fulminant colitis (fever, tachycardia, abdominal pain, toxic megacolon suspicion).
- Severe dehydration or malnutrition.

When to Refer to Specialists (Non-Urgent)

- **Gastroenterology:**
    - ALL suspected IBD.
    - IBS with red flags, refractory symptoms.
- **Dietitian:** IBS or IBD with nutrition issues.
- **Mental health support:** chronic illness burden.

Primary Care Management

- IBS: diagnosis of exclusion, reassurance, lifestyle + symptom management.
- IBD: supportive role, vaccinations, bone health, mental health, cancer screening.
- Monitor for complications (strictures, fistulas, colon cancer in IBD).

Pocket Box – Office IBS vs IBD Quick Reference

- **Step 1:** Chronic abdominal pain + bowel change → consider IBS vs IBD.
- **Step 2:** Red flags → order labs, fecal calprotectin, colonoscopy referral.
- **Step 3:** IBS → lifestyle, low FODMAP, symptom-based meds.
- **Step 4:** IBD → refer GI, support long-term care.

37. Constipation & Diarrhea

Constipation

Definition: <3 bowel movements/week, hard stools, straining.

Causes:

- Functional/slow transit (most common).
- Medications: opioids, anticholinergics, iron, CCBs.
- Metabolic: hypothyroidism, hypercalcemia, diabetes.
- Neurologic: Parkinson's, MS, spinal cord injury.
- Structural: colorectal cancer, strictures.

Investigations (if red flags):

- Red flags: blood in stool, anemia, weight loss, FHx colon cancer, new onset >50.
- Labs: CBC, TSH, calcium.
- Colonoscopy if red flags or refractory.

Management:

- Lifestyle: ↑fiber, fluids, exercise, toileting routine.
- Medications:

- Bulk agents (psyllium).
- Osmotic (PEG, lactulose).
- Stimulant (senna, bisacodyl) short-term.
- Suppositories/enemas for refractory.

Diarrhea

Definition: >3 loose/watery stools/day.

Causes:

- **Acute (<2 weeks):** viral (norovirus, rotavirus), bacterial (Campylobacter, Salmonella, E. coli, C. diff), parasites (Giardia).
- **Chronic (>4 weeks):** IBS, IBD, celiac, lactose intolerance, pancreatic insufficiency, medications (metformin, antibiotics).

Investigations:

- Acute: usually none unless severe/prolonged → stool cultures, C. diff toxin.
- Chronic: CBC, electrolytes, TSH, celiac serology, stool O&P, fecal calprotectin, colonoscopy if red flags.

Management:

- Acute viral: supportive (hydration, electrolytes).
- Bacterial: antibiotics only for severe/prolonged or specific pathogens (e.g., C. diff, Campylobacter).
- Chronic: treat underlying cause (IBS, IBD, celiac, pancreatic enzyme replacement).
- Avoid antimotility drugs if bloody diarrhea/fever (risk of toxic megacolon).

When to Refer to ED (Urgent)

- Severe dehydration, electrolyte imbalance.
- Bloody diarrhea with systemic symptoms.
- Toxic megacolon suspicion (distension, fever, tachycardia, hypotension).
- Severe constipation with obstruction/perforation signs.

When to Refer to Specialists (Non-Urgent)

- GI: chronic diarrhea with red flags, refractory constipation, abnormal colonoscopy findings.
- Dietitian: dietary causes, IBS.

Primary Care Management

- Most acute diarrhea (supportive).
- Functional constipation with lifestyle + laxatives.
- Basic investigations for chronic symptoms.
- Early recognition of red flags and referral.

Pocket Box – Office Constipation/Diarrhea Quick Reference

- **Step 1:** Constipation → rule out meds, red flags → lifestyle + laxatives.
- **Step 2:** Diarrhea → acute (supportive), chronic (screen + targeted therapy).
- **Step 3:** Refer ED if severe dehydration, obstruction, toxic megacolon.

Step 4: GI referral if red flags, refractory, chronic unexplained.

38. Celiac Disease

Definition

- Autoimmune disorder triggered by gluten (wheat, barley, rye).
- Causes villous atrophy in small intestine → malabsorption.

Risk Factors

- Family history of celiac disease.
- Other autoimmune conditions: type 1 diabetes, thyroid disease.
- Down syndrome, Turner syndrome.

Clinical Presentation

- GI: chronic diarrhea, bloating, abdominal pain, weight loss, steatorrhea.
- Extra-intestinal: anemia (iron/folate), osteoporosis, dermatitis herpetiformis, infertility, neuropathy.
- Children: failure to thrive, delayed puberty.

Diagnosis in Office

- Serology: **tTG-IgA** (preferred), total IgA (to exclude deficiency).
- If IgA deficient → deamidated gliadin peptide (DGP) or IgG-based tests.
- Confirm with **small bowel biopsy** (via gastroenterology).
- **Important:** patient must be on a gluten-containing diet for testing.

Initial Office Management

- Counsel **do not start gluten-free diet before testing**.
- If strongly suspected → order serology and refer GI.
- Screen for complications: anemia, vitamin D deficiency, osteoporosis.
- Vaccinations: pneumococcal (if hyposplenism).

Long-Term Management

- Lifelong **gluten-free diet** (dietitian referral essential).
- Nutritional supplementation (iron, folate, vitamin D, calcium, B12).
- Monitor symptoms, serology (tTG-IgA) annually.

- Screen family members if symptomatic or high risk.

When to Refer to ED (Urgent)

- Rare — unless severe dehydration from diarrhea or acute complications.

When to Refer to Specialists (Non-Urgent)

- **Gastroenterology:** ALL suspected cases for biopsy confirmation.
- **Dietitian:** gluten-free diet education.
- **Endocrinology/Hematology:** refractory cases, persistent anemia, bone complications.

Primary Care Management

- Initial suspicion, ordering serology.
- Monitoring adherence and complications once diagnosed.
- Coordinating care with dietitian and gastroenterologist.

Pocket Box – Office Celiac Quick Reference

- **Step 1:** Suspect with chronic diarrhea, anemia, osteoporosis.
- **Step 2:** Order tTG-IgA + total IgA.
- **Step 3:** Refer GI for biopsy confirmation.
- **Step 4:** Gluten-free diet (after diagnosis) + nutritional support.

Step 5: Monitor symptoms, labs annually.

39. Hepatitis B & C

Hepatitis B (HBV)

Transmission: blood, sexual, perinatal.

Screening:

- High-risk groups: immigrants from endemic areas, IV drug use, men who have sex with men, HIV+, household/sexual contacts of HBV carriers, pregnant women.
- Tests: HBsAg, anti-HBs, anti-HBc (total/IgM).

Interpretation:

- HBsAg + → active infection.
- Anti-HBs + only → immune (vaccinated).
- Anti-HBc + + HBsAg − → past infection.

Management (office):

- Acute HBV → supportive.
- Chronic HBV → refer hepatology.
- Vaccinate all non-immune at-risk patients.
- Monitor LFTs, screen for HCC (ultrasound q6mo if cirrhotic).

Hepatitis C (HCV)

Transmission: blood-borne (IV drug use, transfusion pre-1992, tattoos, needle sticks).

Screening:

- Baby boomers (1945–1975), IV drug users, immigrants from endemic regions.
- Test: anti-HCV antibody → if +, confirm with HCV RNA PCR.

Management (office):

- Counsel on transmission (avoid sharing razors, toothbrushes, needles).
- Vaccinate against Hepatitis A & B if not immune.
- Refer ALL confirmed HCV cases to hepatology for direct-acting antivirals (DAAs).
- DAAs cure >95% of cases (8–12 weeks).

Complications of Chronic HBV & HCV

- Cirrhosis, portal hypertension, hepatocellular carcinoma (HCC).

- Extrahepatic: cryoglobulinemia, glomerulonephritis, lymphoma (esp. HCV).

When to Refer to ED (Urgent)

- Acute liver failure: jaundice, coagulopathy, encephalopathy.
- GI bleed from varices.

When to Refer to Specialists (Non-Urgent)

- **Hepatology/Gastroenterology:** ALL chronic HBV/HCV.
- **Infectious diseases:** co-infection with HIV or TB.
- **Oncology:** if HCC detected.

Primary Care Management

- Screen at-risk populations.
- Vaccinate non-immune contacts (HAV, HBV).
- Monitor LFTs, encourage alcohol abstinence.
- Coordinate long-term surveillance (HCC, cirrhosis).

Pocket Box – Office HBV/HCV Quick Reference

- **Step 1:** Screen at-risk groups (HBsAg, anti-HBs, anti-HBc; anti-HCV + PCR).
- **Step 2:** Vaccinate non-immune (HAV/HBV).
- **Step 3:** Refer chronic HBV/HCV to hepatology for treatment.

Step 4: PCP role = screening, vaccination, monitoring, lifestyle counselling.

40. Non-Alcoholic Fatty Liver Disease (NAFLD)

Definition

- Hepatic steatosis (fat in ≥5% of hepatocytes) in absence of significant alcohol use or other causes.
- Spectrum: simple steatosis → NASH (non-alcoholic steatohepatitis) → fibrosis → cirrhosis → HCC.

Risk Factors

- Obesity, metabolic syndrome.
- Type 2 diabetes.
- Dyslipidemia.
- Hypertension.
- Sedentary lifestyle.

Clinical Presentation

- Usually asymptomatic, found incidentally.
- Hepatomegaly, mild RUQ discomfort.
- Often elevated ALT/AST (ALT > AST).

Diagnosis in Office

- History: exclude alcohol (>2 drinks/day men, >1 drink/day women).
- Labs: ALT/AST, ALP, GGT, bilirubin, CBC, glucose, lipids.
- Imaging: ultrasound = first-line (fatty infiltration).
- Fibrosis risk assessment: FIB-4, NAFLD Fibrosis Score.
- Definitive: liver biopsy (specialist).

Initial Office Management

- Lifestyle modification:
    - Weight loss (7–10% reduces steatosis/fibrosis).
    - Diet: Mediterranean/DASH.
    - Physical activity ≥150 min/week.
- Optimize comorbidities:
    - T2DM: consider GLP-1 or SGLT2 inhibitors.
    - Dyslipidemia: statins safe in NAFLD.
    - Hypertension: treat per guidelines.
- Avoid hepatotoxic drugs (monitor if unavoidable).
- Vaccinate HAV, HBV if not immune.

When to Refer to ED (Urgent)

- Acute liver failure: jaundice, coagulopathy, encephalopathy.
- Variceal bleed or decompensated cirrhosis (ascites, encephalopathy, GI bleed).

When to Refer to Specialists (Non-Urgent)

- Hepatology/Gastroenterology if:
  - Uncertain diagnosis.
  - Fibrosis risk (↑FIB-4, elastography abnormal).
  - Cirrhosis or complications.
  - Consideration of biopsy or advanced therapies.

Primary Care Management

- Most mild-moderate NAFLD.
- Lifestyle and comorbidity management.
- Periodic monitoring (LFTs, fibrosis risk scores).
- Vaccinations, alcohol avoidance counselling.

Pocket Box – Office NAFLD Quick Reference

- **Step 1:** Suspect with obesity, diabetes, metabolic syndrome, ↑ALT.
- **Step 2:** Ultrasound + labs to confirm/exclude other causes.
- **Step 3:** Lifestyle modification (weight loss, exercise, diet).
- **Step 4:** Manage comorbidities (DM, HTN, lipids).

Step 5: Refer hepatology if fibrosis, cirrhosis, or unclear diagnosis.

This page has been left intentionally blank

Section 5: Renal & Urology

41. Chronic Kidney Disease (CKD)

Definition

- Abnormal kidney structure or function for ≥3 months.
- **eGFR <60 mL/min/1.73 m²** OR markers of kidney damage (albuminuria, hematuria, structural changes).

Causes

- Diabetes mellitus (most common).
- Hypertension.
- Glomerulonephritis.
- Polycystic kidney disease.
- Obstructive uropathy.
- Medications (NSAIDs, lithium).

Staging (by eGFR)

- G1: ≥90 + evidence of kidney damage.
- G2: 60–89 + evidence of kidney damage.
- G3a: 45–59.

- G3b: 30–44.
- G4: 15–29.
- G5: <15 (kidney failure).

Albuminuria (ACR):

- A1: <3 mg/mmol.
- A2: 3–30.
- A3: >30.

Initial Office Work-Up

- eGFR (serum creatinine, CKD-EPI).
- Urine ACR (albumin-to-creatinine ratio).
- Urinalysis (hematuria, proteinuria).
- BP measurement.
- Additional labs: electrolytes, HbA1c, fasting glucose, lipids, CBC, calcium, phosphate, PTH, vitamin D.
- Renal ultrasound (if hematuria, obstruction, or suspicion of structural disease).

Monitoring

- **Low risk (G1–2, A1):** yearly.
- **Moderate risk (G3a, A2):** every 6 months.

- **High risk (G3b–G5, A3):** every 3 months.

Management in Primary Care

- Optimize comorbidities (diabetes, hypertension, lipids).
- Target BP: <130/80 (use ACEi/ARB if albuminuria).
- Lifestyle: low-sodium diet (<2 g/day), exercise, weight management, smoking cessation.
- Avoid nephrotoxins (NSAIDs, contrast, aminoglycosides).
- Vaccinations: influenza, pneumococcal, hepatitis B (if eGFR <30).

When to Refer to ED (Urgent)

- Severe hyperkalemia.
- Pulmonary edema unresponsive to diuretics.
- Uremic symptoms (pericarditis, encephalopathy).
- Rapid decline in renal function.

When to Refer to Nephrology (Non-Urgent)

- eGFR <30 (G4–5).
- Rapid eGFR decline (>5 mL/min/year).
- Persistent ACR >30.
- Resistant hypertension.
- Hematuria/proteinuria with uncertain cause.
- Suspected hereditary or systemic kidney disease.

Pocket Box – Office CKD Quick Reference

- **Step 1:** Diagnose with eGFR <60 or albuminuria ≥3 for >3 months.
- **Step 2:** Stage by eGFR (G1–5) and ACR (A1–A3).
- **Step 3:** Monitor: yearly (low risk), 6mo (moderate), 3mo (high).
- **Step 4:** Manage BP, diabetes, lifestyle, avoid nephrotoxins.

Step 5: Refer nephrology if eGFR <30, ACR >30, rapid decline, or unclear cause.

42. Hematuria & Proteinuria

Hematuria

Definition: ≥3 RBCs/hpf on microscopy (not dipstick alone).

Causes:

- **Glomerular:** IgA nephropathy, post-infectious GN, lupus nephritis.
- **Non-glomerular:** UTI, nephrolithiasis, BPH, bladder/renal cancer, trauma, anticoagulation.

Initial Office Work-Up:

- Confirm with microscopy (exclude false positives from menstruation, exercise).
- Urinalysis (protein, casts, dysmorphic RBCs).
- Urine culture (rule out infection).
- Serum creatinine/eGFR.
- Renal/bladder ultrasound.
- If >40 yrs or risk factors (smoking, occupational exposure) → consider cystoscopy referral.

Proteinuria

Definition:

- ACR ≥3 mg/mmol (persistent).
- Nephrotic range: >300 mg/mmol (or >3.5 g/day).

Causes:

- **Transient/benign:** fever, exercise, orthostatic proteinuria.
- **Persistent:** diabetic nephropathy, glomerulonephritis, hypertension, CKD.
- **Nephrotic syndrome:** proteinuria + hypoalbuminemia + edema ± hyperlipidemia.

Initial Office Work-Up:

- Urine ACR (confirm on 2–3 samples).
- Urinalysis (casts, hematuria).
- Serum creatinine/eGFR.
- BP, diabetes screening.
- Consider renal ultrasound.

When to Refer to ED (Urgent)

- Gross hematuria with clot retention or urinary obstruction.
- Severe nephrotic syndrome with anasarca, thrombosis, or AKI.
- Rapidly progressive renal failure.

When to Refer to Specialists (Non-Urgent)

- **Nephrology:**
  - Persistent proteinuria (ACR >30).
  - Nephrotic syndrome.
  - Hematuria with proteinuria or impaired renal function.
- **Urology:**
  - Gross hematuria (after ruling out infection).
  - Microscopic hematuria with risk factors for malignancy.

Primary Care Management

- Rule out benign/transient causes.
- Monitor mild isolated hematuria without risk factors.
- Manage risk factors: diabetes, hypertension, avoid nephrotoxins.
- Early referral if persistent or unexplained.

Pocket Box – Office Hematuria & Proteinuria Quick Reference

- **Hematuria:** confirm with microscopy → rule out UTI → ultrasound ± cystoscopy.
- **Proteinuria:** confirm with ACR → repeat → screen for DM/HTN/CKD.
- **Refer nephrology:** persistent proteinuria, nephrotic syndrome, renal dysfunction.

Refer urology: gross hematuria, high-risk microscopic hematuria.

43. Benign Prostatic Hyperplasia (BPH) & Prostatitis

Benign Prostatic Hyperplasia (BPH)

Clinical Presentation:

- LUTS (lower urinary tract symptoms): hesitancy, weak stream, dribbling, nocturia, frequency, urgency, incomplete emptying.
- Complications: urinary retention, recurrent UTIs, bladder stones, hydronephrosis.

Diagnosis in Office:

- History + IPSS (symptom score).
- DRE: enlarged, smooth prostate.
- Urinalysis (exclude infection/hematuria).
- Serum creatinine (if obstruction suspected).
- PSA (if indicated by age/risk, not mandatory for LUTS alone).

Management:

- Mild symptoms: watchful waiting, lifestyle (reduce fluids at night, avoid caffeine/alcohol).
- Pharmacologic:
    - α-blockers (tamsulosin).
    - 5-α-reductase inhibitors (finasteride) if large prostate.
    - Combination therapy if severe.
- Surgery (TURP, laser) if refractory, retention, recurrent infections, renal impairment.

Prostatitis

Types:

- **Acute bacterial prostatitis:** fever, dysuria, perineal pain, tender boggy prostate.
- **Chronic bacterial prostatitis:** recurrent UTIs, pelvic discomfort.
- **Chronic pelvic pain syndrome:** pelvic pain without infection.

Diagnosis:

- Urinalysis, urine culture.
- Avoid prostatic massage in acute prostatitis (risk of bacteremia).
- Blood cultures if septic.

Management:

- **Acute bacterial:**
    - Ciprofloxacin or TMP-SMX × 4–6 weeks.
    - Hospitalize + IV antibiotics if severe.
- **Chronic bacterial:** prolonged antibiotics (fluoroquinolone × 6–12 weeks).
- **Chronic pelvic pain:** α-blockers, NSAIDs, physiotherapy, supportive care.

When to Refer to ED (Urgent)

- Acute urinary retention.
- Acute prostatitis with sepsis.
- BPH with renal failure or obstructive uropathy.

When to Refer to Specialists (Non-Urgent)

- **Urology:**
    - Refractory or severe BPH (surgical candidates).
    - Recurrent urinary retention.
    - Persistent hematuria.
    - Chronic/recurrent prostatitis not responding to therapy.

Primary Care Management

- Mild/moderate BPH with α-blockers/5-ARIs.
- Uncomplicated prostatitis with antibiotics.
- Monitoring PSA (if indicated), renal function, symptoms.

Pocket Box – Office BPH/Prostatitis Quick Reference

- **BPH:** LUTS + DRE → lifestyle, α-blocker ± 5-ARI → refer if refractory/complicated.

Prostatitis: fever, dysuria, tender prostate → antibiotics × 4–6 wks → ED if septic or obstructed.

44. Urinary Tract Infections (UTIs): Pediatric, Male, Female & Recurrent

Definition

- Infection of urinary tract: cystitis, pyelonephritis, asymptomatic bacteriuria (ASB).

UTIs in Women

Presentation: dysuria, frequency, urgency, suprapubic pain, hematuria.
Diagnosis: urinalysis (leukocyte esterase, nitrite, pyuria), urine culture if complicated or recurrent.
Management:

- Uncomplicated cystitis: nitrofurantoin × 5 days, TMP-SMX × 3 days, fosfomycin single dose.
- Pyelonephritis: ciprofloxacin × 7 days or ceftriaxone IV then oral step-down.
ASB: treat only if pregnant or before urologic procedures.

UTIs in Men

- Always considered **complicated**.
- Rule out prostatitis or obstruction (BPH).
- Antibiotics: fluoroquinolones or TMP-SMX × 7–14 days (adjust to culture).
- Investigate recurrent UTIs (renal/bladder ultrasound, post-void residual).

Pediatric UTIs

Presentation:

- Infants: fever, irritability, poor feeding, vomiting.
- Older children: dysuria, frequency, abdominal pain.
  Work-up:
- Urine culture (catheter or clean-catch).
- Renal/bladder ultrasound after first febrile UTI in <2 yrs.
- VCUG if recurrent or abnormal ultrasound.
  Management:
- Oral cefixime, TMP-SMX, or amoxicillin-clavulanate (based on local resistance).
- IV antibiotics (ceftriaxone, gentamicin) if toxic/septic.

Recurrent UTIs

- ≥2 infections in 6 months OR ≥3 in 12 months.
- Risk factors: sexual activity, spermicide use, postmenopause, anatomic abnormalities.
- Management:
    - Behavioural: hydration, post-coital voiding, avoid spermicides.
    - Vaginal estrogen in postmenopausal women.
    - Prophylactic antibiotics (continuous or post-coital) if frequent recurrences.
    - Investigate anatomic/functional abnormalities if persistent.

When to Refer to ED (Urgent)

- Urosepsis (fever, hypotension, tachycardia).
- Acute pyelonephritis with systemic illness.
- Urinary retention with infection.

When to Refer to Specialists (Non-Urgent)

- Recurrent UTIs despite prophylaxis.
- Suspected structural abnormality.
- Pediatric recurrent febrile UTIs.
- Male UTIs with obstruction or prostatitis.

Primary Care Management

- Diagnose and treat uncomplicated female cystitis.
- Manage most pediatric and male UTIs if mild and straightforward.
- Screen and treat ASB in pregnancy only.
- Counsel on prevention strategies.

Pocket Box – Office UTI Quick Reference

- **Women:** dysuria/frequency → nitrofurantoin 5d, TMP-SMX 3d.
- **Men:** always complicated → 7–14d abx, investigate.
- **Kids:** urine culture, ultrasound if <2 yrs febrile UTI.
- **Recurrent:** behavioural + prophylaxis ± urology referral.

Refer ED: sepsis, pyelonephritis, obstruction.

45. Nephrolithiasis (Kidney Stones)

Definition

- Formation of crystalline stones in urinary tract (calcium oxalate most common).

Risk Factors

- Dehydration (low fluid intake, hot climate).
- High sodium, high oxalate, high animal protein diet.
- Hyperparathyroidism, gout, RTA, obesity, diabetes.
- Family history, prior stones.

Clinical Presentation

- Flank pain → severe, colicky, radiates to groin/testicle/labia.
- Hematuria (gross or microscopic).
- Nausea, vomiting.
- Dysuria, urgency if distal ureter involved.

Diagnosis in Office/ED

- Urinalysis: hematuria, crystals, infection signs.
- Serum: creatinine, calcium, uric acid, electrolytes.
- Imaging:
    - Non-contrast CT abdomen/pelvis = gold standard.
    - Ultrasound: preferred in pregnancy, useful for hydronephrosis.
    - KUB X-ray: limited (only radio-opaque stones).

Management

In Primary Care / Office Setting

- Pain control: NSAIDs (first-line), acetaminophen, opioids if severe.
- Encourage oral hydration (unless obstructed).
- Tamsulosin for medical expulsive therapy if distal stone <10 mm.
- Advise urine straining for stone analysis.
- Arrange outpatient imaging if not done in ED.
- Antibiotics if UTI suspected.

When to Refer to ED (Urgent)

- Fever + obstruction (urologic emergency, risk of sepsis).
- Anuria or bilateral obstruction.
- AKI or rising creatinine with obstruction.
- Uncontrolled pain or vomiting preventing oral intake.

When to Refer to Specialists (Non-Urgent)

- Stones >10 mm or not passed after 4–6 weeks.
- Recurrent stones.
- Anatomical abnormalities.
- Pediatric nephrolithiasis.

Prevention & Long-Term Care

- Fluid intake to produce ≥2.5 L urine/day.
- Reduce sodium and animal protein.
- Avoid excessive oxalate (spinach, nuts, chocolate).
- Maintain adequate dietary calcium (do not restrict too much).
- Consider thiazides, allopurinol, or potassium citrate for recurrent stone formers (per specialist guidance).

Pocket Box – Office Nephrolithiasis Quick Reference

- **Step 1:** Flank pain + hematuria → UA + imaging.
- **Step 2:** Manage in office: NSAIDs, fluids, tamsulosin, strain urine.
- **Step 3:** Refer ED if fever + obstruction, AKI, uncontrolled pain.
- **Step 4:** Refer urology if >10 mm, non-passage, or recurrent.

Step 5: Counsel on prevention: hydration, diet, metabolic work-up if recurrent.

This page has been left intentionally blank

Section 6: Women's Health

46. Contraception Overview

Types of Contraception

- **Short-acting hormonal:**
    - Combined oral contraceptives (COCs): estrogen + progestin.
    - Progestin-only pill (POP).
    - Patch, vaginal ring.
- **Long-acting reversible contraception (LARC):**
    - Progestin implant (not widely available in Canada).
    - Progestin IUD (levonorgestrel).
    - Copper IUD.
- **Barrier methods:** male/female condoms, diaphragm, cervical cap.
- **Other:** withdrawal (least reliable), fertility awareness.
- **Permanent:** tubal ligation, vasectomy (for partners).

Efficacy (Typical Use Failure Rates)

- LARC (<1%).
- Pills, patch, ring (~7%).
- Condoms (13–21%).
- Withdrawal (~20%).

Office / Primary Care Management

- **Assessment:** medical history (contraindications, comorbidities, smoking, migraine, VTE risk).
- **Counselling:**
    - Effectiveness, side effects, reversibility.
    - STI protection only with condoms.
- **Prescribing:**
    - COC: avoid if smoker >35 yrs, migraine with aura, VTE history, uncontrolled HTN.
    - POP: suitable if estrogen contraindicated, breastfeeding.
    - IUD: highly effective; offer as first-line for adolescents and nulliparous as well.
- **Monitoring:**
    - Check BP with COCs.
    - Review side effects, adherence.

When to Refer to ED (Urgent)

- Suspected VTE (DVT/PE).
- Stroke or MI symptoms.
- Severe migraine with neurologic deficit after starting COC.
- Sepsis after IUD insertion (rare).

When to Refer to Specialists (Non-Urgent)

- Gynecology:
    - Complex medical comorbidities and contraception needs.
    - Difficulty with IUD insertion or complications (perforation, expulsion).
    - Desire for sterilization (tubal ligation).
- Hematology: thrombophilia evaluation if strong FHx of clotting.

Long-Term / Prevention

- Encourage dual protection (condoms + hormonal/IUD) for STI and pregnancy prevention.
- Reassess contraception choice regularly (age, comorbidities, fertility plans).
- Counsel on return of fertility after stopping.
- Ensure regular preventive care (Pap smear, STI screening, vaccinations).

Pocket Box – Office Contraception Quick Reference

- **Step 1:** Assess contraindications (smoking >35, VTE, migraine with aura).
- **Step 2:** Discuss options → prioritize LARC for best efficacy.
- **Step 3:** Prescribe COC/POP/patch/ring if safe; offer condoms for STI protection.
- **Step 4:** Refer ED if VTE/stroke/MI suspected.

Step 5: Refer gynecology for complex cases or sterilization.

47. Menstrual Disorders (Dysmenorrhea, Abnormal Bleeding, Amenorrhea)

Dysmenorrhea

- **Primary:** painful periods without pelvic pathology (common in adolescents).
- **Secondary:** due to endometriosis, adenomyosis, fibroids, PID.
- **Office Management:**
    - NSAIDs (first-line, start before onset).
    - Combined OCPs or hormonal IUD for cycle control.
    - Lifestyle: exercise, heat therapy.

Abnormal Uterine Bleeding (AUB)

- **PALM-COEIN classification:**
    - Structural: Polyps, Adenomyosis, Leiomyoma, Malignancy.
    - Non-structural: Coagulopathy, Ovulatory dysfunction,

Endometrial, Iatrogenic, Not otherwise classified.
- **Initial Work-up in Office:**
    - History (cycle, flow, bleeding risk).
    - Exam (pelvic exam, Pap if due).
    - Labs: CBC, TSH, pregnancy test, STI screen if indicated.
    - Pelvic ultrasound.
- **Management in Office:**
    - Acute heavy bleeding: high-dose combined OCP or progestin.
    - Chronic management: COC, levonorgestrel IUD, tranexamic acid, NSAIDs.

Amenorrhea

- **Primary:** no menarche by age 15 (or 13 without secondary sexual characteristics).
- **Secondary:** absence of menses ≥3 months (previously regular) or ≥6 months (previously irregular).
- **Initial Work-up in Office:**
    - Pregnancy test (always first).
    - TSH, prolactin, FSH/LH, estradiol.
    - Consider PCOS (history, ultrasound, labs).

- Assess eating disorders, exercise, stress.
- **Management in Office:**
  - Treat underlying cause (thyroid disease, hyperprolactinemia, PCOS).
  - Hormonal therapy for cycle regulation (OCPs, progestins).
  - Counsel on bone health if prolonged hypoestrogenism.

When to Refer to ED (Urgent)

- Hemodynamically unstable bleeding (soaking pads hourly, symptomatic anemia).
- Severe pain with suspected ovarian torsion or ruptured ectopic pregnancy.

When to Refer to Specialists (Non-Urgent)

- Gynecology:
  - AUB not responding to initial therapy.
  - Structural pathology (fibroids, polyps, suspected malignancy).
  - Primary amenorrhea, complex secondary amenorrhea, suspected PCOS/POI.

- Endocrinology: hypothalamic/pituitary disorders.
- Hematology: suspected bleeding disorder.

Long-Term / Prevention

- Regular follow-up for response to therapy.
- Screen for anemia in chronic heavy bleeding.
- Bone health monitoring in chronic amenorrhea.
- Contraceptive counselling as part of menstrual management.

Pocket Box – Office Menstrual Disorders Quick Reference

- **Dysmenorrhea:** NSAIDs ± OCP/hormonal IUD.
- **AUB:** CBC, TSH, pelvic US → OCP, LNG-IUD, tranexamic acid.
- **Amenorrhea:** rule out pregnancy → TSH, prolactin, FSH/LH → treat cause.
- **Refer ED:** unstable bleeding, torsion/ectopic.

Refer Gyn: refractory bleeding, structural cause, amenorrhea work-up.

48. Antenatal & Postnatal Care in Family Practice

Antenatal Care (Routine Pregnancy Care in Primary Care)

- **Initial Visit (ideally <12 weeks):**
    - History: obstetric, medical, family, social, medications.
    - Physical: BP, BMI, pelvic exam if indicated.
    - Labs: CBC, blood type + antibody screen, rubella, hepatitis B, HIV, syphilis, urine culture, varicella immunity, HbA1c if risk factors.
    - Folic acid supplementation (0.4–1 mg/day; 5 mg/day if high risk).
- **Ongoing Visits:**
    - Every 4 weeks until 28 wks → every 2 wks until 36 wks → weekly until delivery.
    - Monitor BP, weight, urine dip (protein), fundal height, fetal heart.
- **Screening:**
    - Gestational diabetes: 24–28 wks (50 g GTT).
    - GBS swab: 35–37 wks.

- o Ultrasound: dating (≤12 wks), anatomy (18–22 wks), growth if indicated.
- **Vaccinations:**
  - o Tdap at 27–32 wks.
  - o Influenza vaccine if in season.
- **Counselling:** nutrition, exercise, smoking/alcohol cessation, warning signs (bleeding, decreased fetal movement, preeclampsia).

Postnatal Care (Mother & Infant)

- **Maternal:**
  - o Assess bleeding, wound healing (C-section, episiotomy).
  - o Screen for postpartum depression (EPDS).
  - o Contraceptive counselling (LARC, POP safe in breastfeeding).
  - o Counsel on lactation, sleep, support.
- **Infant:**
  - o Feeding assessment (breast/bottle).
  - o Growth and development monitoring.
  - o Vaccinations per schedule.
  - o Screen for jaundice, congenital hip dysplasia, cardiac issues.

When to Refer to ED (Urgent)

- Pregnancy: vaginal bleeding, ruptured membranes, preeclampsia symptoms, reduced fetal movement, preterm labour.
- Postpartum: heavy hemorrhage, infection (endometritis, wound sepsis), severe depression or psychosis, thromboembolism.
- Neonatal: poor feeding, lethargy, fever, jaundice <24 hrs, respiratory distress.

When to Refer to Specialists (Non-Urgent)

- **Obstetrics:** high-risk pregnancy (multiple gestation, preeclampsia, gestational diabetes requiring insulin, fetal growth restriction).
- **Psychiatry:** postpartum depression/psychosis not manageable in primary care.
- **Lactation consultant/pediatrics:** feeding difficulties, failure to thrive.

Long-Term / Prevention

- Ongoing maternal health: BP, diabetes screening, contraception, Pap test.

- Support breastfeeding for ≥6 months if possible.
- Encourage healthy sleep, nutrition, physical activity postpartum.
- Mental health support and community resources.

Pocket Box – Office Antenatal & Postnatal Quick Reference

- **Step 1:** Initial visit labs, folic acid, counselling.
- **Step 2:** Routine follow-ups (4wks → 2wks → weekly).
- **Step 3:** Screen GDM (24–28 wks), GBS (35–37 wks).
- **Step 4:** Postpartum: bleeding, mood, contraception, infant feeding/growth.

Step 5: Refer ED if hemorrhage, preeclampsia, sepsis, neonatal distress.

49. Menopause & Hormone Replacement Therapy (HRT)

Definition

- **Menopause:** 12 months of amenorrhea after final menstrual period (average age 51).
- **Perimenopause:** transition period with irregular cycles and menopausal symptoms.

Clinical Features

- Vasomotor: hot flashes, night sweats.
- Genitourinary: vaginal dryness, dyspareunia, recurrent UTIs.
- Mood/cognitive: irritability, insomnia, memory changes.
- Long-term: osteoporosis, ↑ cardiovascular risk.

Office / Primary Care Management

- **Lifestyle & Support:**
    - Exercise, weight management, sleep hygiene.

- o Limit caffeine, alcohol, smoking cessation.
- **Vasomotor symptoms:**
  - o 1st line: HRT if no contraindications.
  - o Alternatives (if HRT contraindicated): SSRIs (paroxetine, venlafaxine), gabapentin, clonidine.
- **Genitourinary syndrome:**
  - o Vaginal estrogen (cream, tablet, ring).
  - o Lubricants, moisturizers.
- **Bone health:**
  - o Calcium + vitamin D, weight-bearing exercise.
  - o Bisphosphonates if osteoporosis diagnosed.

HRT (Hormone Replacement Therapy)

- **Indications:** moderate-severe vasomotor or GSM (genitourinary syndrome of menopause).
- **Formulations:**
  - o Estrogen alone (if hysterectomy).
  - o Estrogen + progestin (if uterus intact, to prevent endometrial cancer).

- **Contraindications:** breast/endometrial cancer, unexplained vaginal bleeding, active VTE, CAD, stroke, severe liver disease.
- **Duration:** lowest effective dose, shortest duration (typically <5 years), reassess yearly.

When to Refer to ED (Urgent)

- Suspected VTE, MI, or stroke in patient on HRT.
- Severe uncontrolled bleeding on therapy.

When to Refer to Specialists (Non-Urgent)

- Gynecology: complex cases, contraindications to standard HRT, refractory symptoms.
- Endocrinology: difficult osteoporosis management.
- Psychiatry: severe mood disturbances related to menopause.

Long-Term / Prevention

- Encourage regular physical activity, balanced diet.
- Screen for osteoporosis, CVD risk.
- Mammography as per guidelines.
- Annual reassessment of need for HRT.

Pocket Box – Office Menopause/HRT Quick Reference

- **Step 1:** Diagnose clinically (amenorrhea ≥12 months, symptoms).
- **Step 2:** Lifestyle + reassurance.
- **Step 3:** Offer HRT if moderate-severe symptoms, no contraindications.
- **Step 4:** Vaginal estrogen for GSM, bisphosphonates for osteoporosis.

Step 5: Refer ED if VTE/stroke/MI; refer Gyn if complex or refractory.

50. Breast Disorders (Mastitis, Fibroadenoma, Cancer Screening)

Mastitis

- **Presentation:** localized breast pain, erythema, swelling, fever, malaise.
- **Causes:** most common in lactating women (Staph aureus).
- **Office Management:**
    - Continue breastfeeding/pumping (do not stop).
    - Supportive: analgesia, warm compresses.
    - Antibiotics: cephalexin, cloxacillin, or clindamycin (10–14 days).
- **Complication:** abscess (requires drainage).

Fibroadenoma

- **Presentation:** benign, smooth, mobile, firm breast lump.
- **Diagnosis:**

        - Triple assessment: clinical exam, imaging (US or mammogram if >30 yrs), biopsy/FNA.
- **Office Management:**
    - Reassurance if benign confirmed.
    - Monitor with imaging if <3 cm and stable.
    - Surgical excision if large, growing, or bothersome.

Breast Cancer Screening (Canadian Guidelines)

- **Average-risk women:**
    - Ages 50–74: mammogram every 2 years.
    - Ages 40–49: discuss risks/benefits, individualized decision.
    - 74: case-by-case depending on life expectancy.
- **High-risk women:**
    - BRCA mutation, strong FHx, prior chest radiation → start at 30 with annual MRI + mammogram.

When to Refer to ED (Urgent)

- Severe mastitis with sepsis.
- Breast abscess with systemic illness.

When to Refer to Specialists (Non-Urgent)

- **General Surgery / Breast Specialist:**
    - Suspicious lump or abnormal imaging.
    - Abscess requiring drainage.
    - Recurrent mastitis or persistent symptoms.
- **Genetics:** strong FHx of breast/ovarian cancer.
- **Oncology:** confirmed malignancy.

Long-Term / Prevention

- Encourage breast self-awareness (not formal self-exam).
- Promote breastfeeding (reduces breast cancer risk).
- Counsel on screening adherence.
- Lifestyle: exercise, healthy weight, limit alcohol.

Pocket Box – Office Breast Disorders Quick Reference

- **Mastitis:** continue breastfeeding + antibiotics → refer if abscess/sepsis.
- **Fibroadenoma:** smooth, mobile lump → triple assessment → reassure/monitor.
- **Screening:** 50–74 mammogram q2y; earlier if high risk.

Refer: suspicious lump, abnormal imaging, abscess.

Section 7: Men's Health

51. Prostate Health (BPH, Cancer Screening)

Benign Prostatic Hyperplasia (BPH)

- **Symptoms:** LUTS (frequency, urgency, nocturia, hesitancy, weak stream, dribbling, incomplete emptying).
- **Complications:** urinary retention, recurrent UTIs, bladder stones, hydronephrosis, renal impairment.

Office / Primary Care Management

- History: LUTS assessment (IPSS score).
- Exam: DRE (smooth, enlarged prostate).
- Labs: urinalysis (exclude infection/hematuria), creatinine (if obstruction suspected).
- PSA: optional, only if result would change management (not for LUTS alone).
- Mild symptoms → watchful waiting, lifestyle: reduce evening fluids, avoid caffeine/alcohol, timed voiding.
- Moderate-severe symptoms → α-blocker (tamsulosin); 5-ARI

(finasteride) if large prostate; combination if severe.

When to Refer to ED (Urgent)

- Acute urinary retention.
- Obstructive uropathy with renal failure.
- Sepsis with urinary obstruction.

When to Refer to Specialists (Non-Urgent)

- Urology: refractory LUTS, recurrent retention, gross hematuria, suspicion of prostate/bladder cancer, complications (stones, hydronephrosis).

Prostate Cancer Screening

Epidemiology: most common male cancer; risk increases with age, family history, African ancestry.

Screening (Canadian guidance):

- Routine population screening **not recommended**.
- **Shared decision-making**:
    - Men 55–69 may opt for PSA screening after counselling on risks/benefits.
    - Not recommended <55 or >70 unless high risk.

Office / Primary Care Management

- Discuss pros/cons of PSA (overdiagnosis, overtreatment vs mortality benefit).
- If PSA ordered:
    - Normal range depends on age.
    - DRE: hard, nodular, asymmetry → suspicious.
- Repeat PSA if borderline before referral.

When to Refer to ED (Urgent)

- Rare; only if spinal cord compression symptoms (back pain, neuro deficits) in known prostate cancer.

When to Refer to Specialists (Non-Urgent)

- Urology: abnormal DRE, persistently elevated PSA, strong FHx with concern.

Long-Term / Prevention

- Encourage healthy weight, exercise, balanced diet.
- Regular follow-up of LUTS and PSA if opted.
- In cancer survivors: monitor for recurrence, side effects of androgen deprivation therapy.

Pocket Box – Office Prostate Health Quick Reference

- **BPH:** LUTS + DRE → lifestyle/α-blocker → refer if retention, hematuria, complications.
- **Prostate Cancer:** discuss PSA pros/cons (55–69 yrs) → refer urology if abnormal DRE or persistently high PSA.

Refer ED: retention, renal failure, sepsis, cord compression.

52. Erectile Dysfunction (ED)

Definition

- Persistent inability to achieve or maintain an erection sufficient for satisfactory sexual performance.

Causes

- **Vascular:** atherosclerosis, hypertension, diabetes, smoking.
- **Neurologic:** spinal cord injury, MS, neuropathy.
- **Endocrine:** hypogonadism, thyroid disease, hyperprolactinemia.
- **Medications:** SSRIs, antihypertensives (β-blockers, thiazides), antipsychotics.
- **Psychogenic:** depression, anxiety, relationship issues.

Office / Primary Care Management

- **History:** sexual function, onset, nocturnal erections, comorbidities, meds, psychosocial context.

- **Physical:** BP, BMI, CV exam, genital exam, DRE if indicated.
- **Investigations:** fasting glucose/HbA1c, lipids, testosterone (AM sample), TSH, prolactin if indicated.
- **Lifestyle interventions:** exercise, weight loss, smoking cessation, limit alcohol.
- **Pharmacologic:**
    - PDE5 inhibitors (sildenafil, tadalafil) – contraindicated with nitrates.
    - Dose before sexual activity (sildenafil) or daily/longer duration (tadalafil).
- **Psychological:** counselling, CBT, sex therapy if psychogenic.

When to Refer to ED (Urgent)

- Priapism (erection >4 hours, painful).
- Sudden-onset ED with neurologic symptoms (possible stroke, spinal cord lesion).

When to Refer to Specialists (Non-Urgent)

- **Urology:** failure of PDE5 inhibitors, Peyronie's disease, penile prosthesis consideration.
- **Endocrinology:** hypogonadism, abnormal testosterone/prolactin.
- **Cardiology:** ED with high CV risk before starting PDE5i.
- **Psychiatry/therapy:** psychogenic ED not improving with basic counselling.

Long-Term / Prevention

- Manage underlying cardiovascular risk factors (ED = early marker of CVD).
- Encourage healthy lifestyle, regular exercise, weight management.
- Monitor testosterone levels if on replacement therapy.
- Patient education: avoid unregulated supplements.

Pocket Box – Office ED Quick Reference

- **Step 1:** Assess causes (vascular, neuro, endocrine, meds, psychogenic).
- **Step 2:** Labs (glucose, lipids, testosterone, TSH).

- **Step 3:** Lifestyle + PDE5i (if no nitrates).
- **Step 4:** Refer ED if priapism or sudden neuro deficit.

Step 5: Refer urology/endocrine/cardiology if refractory or complex.

53. Hypogonadism

Definition

- Failure of testes to produce normal testosterone ± sperm due to testicular (primary) or pituitary-hypothalamic (secondary) dysfunction.

Causes

- **Primary (testicular):** Klinefelter syndrome, orchitis (mumps, HIV), trauma, chemotherapy/radiation, aging.
- **Secondary (pituitary/hypothalamic):** pituitary tumors, hyperprolactinemia, chronic illness, obesity, medications (opioids, glucocorticoids).
- **Functional:** obesity, metabolic syndrome, type 2 diabetes, stress.

Clinical Features

- Sexual: decreased libido, erectile dysfunction, infertility.

- Physical: reduced muscle mass, increased fat, decreased shaving frequency, gynecomastia, small testes.
- Systemic: low energy, depression, osteoporosis/low bone density, anemia.

Office / Primary Care Management

- **History:** symptoms of low testosterone, infertility, meds, systemic illness.
- **Physical exam:** body hair, gynecomastia, testicular size, BMI.
- **Investigations:**
    - Morning total testosterone × 2 (low on both = diagnostic).
    - LH/FSH to differentiate primary vs secondary.
    - Prolactin, TSH if secondary suspected.
    - DEXA if osteoporosis suspected.
- **Initial management:**
    - Lifestyle: weight reduction, exercise, optimize sleep, treat comorbidities.
    - Consider endocrinology referral before starting testosterone.
    - Discuss fertility plans (testosterone therapy suppresses spermatogenesis).

When to Refer to ED (Urgent)

- Pituitary apoplexy (sudden headache, vision loss, hypotension).
- Severe symptomatic hypogonadism with acute adrenal or pituitary crisis suspicion.

When to Refer to Specialists (Non-Urgent)

- **Endocrinology:**
    - Confirmed low testosterone on repeat testing.
    - Suspected pituitary/hypothalamic disorder.
    - Initiation/monitoring of testosterone therapy.
- **Urology:** infertility management.
- **Hematology:** unexplained polycythemia on testosterone therapy.

Long-Term / Prevention

- If on testosterone therapy:
    - Monitor CBC, PSA, LFTs, testosterone levels q6–12 months.
    - Counsel on risks: polycythemia, infertility, possible CV events, prostate effects.

- Bone health: calcium, vitamin D, weight-bearing exercise.
- Manage metabolic syndrome/CVD risk factors.

Pocket Box – Office Hypogonadism Quick Reference

- **Step 1:** Suspect with low libido, ED, fatigue, infertility.
- **Step 2:** Morning testosterone ×2 + LH/FSH, prolactin, TSH.
- **Step 3:** Lifestyle + address comorbidities.
- **Step 4:** Refer endocrinology before starting testosterone.

Step 5: Monitor CBC, PSA, testosterone if on therapy.

This page has been left intentionally blank

Section 8: Pediatrics

54. Well Child Care & Immunizations

Introduction

Well child care is one of the cornerstones of family medicine. It provides an opportunity to monitor growth and development, promote preventive health, address parental concerns, and deliver immunizations. Family physicians are uniquely positioned to provide continuity from newborn care through adolescence.

Growth & Development

- **Growth Monitoring:**
    - Plot weight, length/height, head circumference, and BMI at each visit.
    - Use WHO charts <2 yrs; CDC charts >2 yrs.
    - Watch for **crossing percentiles**, failure to thrive, or obesity trends.
- **Developmental Surveillance:**
    - Domains: **gross motor, fine motor, speech/language, social/adaptive**.

- Use validated tools if concerns: Ages & Stages Questionnaire (ASQ), M-CHAT (autism screen at 18–24 months).
- Red flags: loss of milestones, no social smile by 3 months, not sitting by 9 months, not walking by 18 months, not talking by 2 years.

Nutrition & Feeding

- **Infants:**
    - Exclusive breastfeeding to 6 months recommended; continue with solids to 2 years and beyond.
    - Vitamin D 400 IU/day for all breastfed infants.
    - Formula: use iron-fortified; vitamin D not required.
    - Introduce solids ~6 months (iron-rich: fortified cereal, meats, legumes).
    - Allergenic foods (peanut, egg, fish) should be introduced early (before 1 year) unless contraindicated.
- **Toddlers/Children:**
    - Encourage family meals, varied diet.

- o Limit juice (≤125 mL/day if given at all).
- o Avoid sugar-sweetened beverages.
- **Adolescents:**
  - o Counsel on body image, healthy eating.
  - o Screen for eating disorders if concerns (amenorrhea, rapid weight loss, restrictive eating).
  - o Monitor iron intake (menstruating females at risk for deficiency).

Sleep & Safety

- **Infants:**
  - o Back to sleep, own crib/bassinet, firm mattress, no soft bedding.
  - o Room sharing recommended for first 6 months.
- **Toddlers/Children:**
  - o Consistent bedtime routines.
  - o Discuss nightmares, night terrors, sleep hygiene.
- **Adolescents:**
  - o Screen for sleep deprivation, screen time, late-night device use.
- **Safety Counselling:**

- Car seats: rear-facing until ≥2 yrs, then forward-facing → booster → seatbelt.
- Bicycle/skating: helmets always.
- Home safety: gates, window guards, safe storage of medications/cleaning products, water safety.
- Adolescents: substance use, peer pressure, safe sex, driving safety.

Immunizations (Canadian Schedule – Key Highlights)

- **Routine Childhood Vaccines:**
    - 2, 4, 6 months: DTaP-IPV-Hib, PCV, rotavirus.
    - 12 months: MMR, varicella, meningococcal, hepatitis A (some provinces).
    - 15–18 months: DTaP-IPV-Hib booster, MMRV.
    - 4–6 years: DTaP-IPV, MMRV boosters.
- **Adolescent Vaccines:**
    - HPV (Grade 6–7, 2-dose series if <15 yrs, 3-dose if older).
    - Tdap booster at 14–16 yrs.
    - Meningococcal (Men-C or Men-ACYW).

- o Annual influenza vaccine.
- **Special Populations:**
  - o Preterm infants: follow chronological age, not corrected age.
  - o Immunocompromised: avoid live vaccines (MMR, varicella).
  - o High-risk: hepatitis B, meningococcal, influenza yearly.

Office / Primary Care Management

- **Schedule of Visits:**
  - o Newborn, 2 wks, 2, 4, 6, 9, 12, 15, 18 months, then annually.
- **Components of Each Visit:**
  - o Growth & development monitoring.
  - o Anticipatory guidance (nutrition, sleep, safety, parenting).
  - o Physical exam tailored to age.
  - o Immunizations as per schedule.
  - o Address parental concerns (feeding, sleep, behaviour, milestones).
- **Screening in Primary Care:**
  - o Vision screening by age 3–5 yrs.
  - o Hearing screening (newborn, preschool).

    - Anemia screening if risk factors.
    - Lead/TB if environmental or epidemiological risk.

When to Refer to ED (Urgent)

- Febrile infant <2 months.
- Severe vaccine reaction (anaphylaxis, hypotonia-hyporesponsive episode).
- Child with growth failure and systemic illness.
- Respiratory distress or dehydration during well-child check.

When to Refer to Specialists (Non-Urgent)

- **Pediatrics:** developmental delay, failure to thrive, complex behavioural issues.
- **Immunology/Infectious Disease:** suspected vaccine contraindications, recurrent infections.
- **Endocrinology/Genetics:** growth abnormalities.
- **ENT/Audiology:** confirmed hearing loss.
- **Ophthalmology:** strabismus, failed vision screening.

Long-Term / Prevention

- Reinforce healthy lifestyle at every visit (nutrition, physical activity, mental health).
- Promote school readiness, positive parenting, social support.
- Ensure vaccine adherence to prevent outbreaks.
- Encourage safe technology use (screen time limits).

Pocket Box – Office Well Child Care Quick Reference

- **Step 1:** Growth & developmental monitoring every visit.
- **Step 2:** Breastfeeding to 6 months; solids at 6 months; vitamin D.
- **Step 3:** Sleep safety: back to sleep, own crib, no soft bedding.
- **Step 4:** Safety counselling: car seats, helmets, poison-proofing.
- **Step 5:** Vaccinate per Canadian schedule; flu yearly.

Step 6: Refer ED for febrile infant <2mo, vaccine reaction; refer peds for developmental or growth concerns.

55. Common Pediatric Infections

Introduction

Infections are the most common reason for pediatric visits in family practice. Most are viral and self-limited, but distinguishing benign illness from serious bacterial infection is essential. Family physicians provide diagnosis, reassurance, symptomatic care, and early recognition of complications.

Acute Otitis Media (AOM)

- **Presentation:** fever, irritability, ear pain, pulling at ear, URI symptoms.
- **Exam:** bulging, erythematous tympanic membrane with decreased mobility.
- **Office Management:**
    - Pain control: acetaminophen, ibuprofen.
    - Watchful waiting (≥ 6 months, mild symptoms, unilateral).
    - Antibiotics: amoxicillin (first-line) 80–90 mg/kg/day × 10 days.

- **When to Refer ED:** mastoiditis (post-auricular swelling, redness), meningitis symptoms, sepsis.
- **When to Refer Specialists:** ENT for recurrent AOM (≥3 in 6 months or ≥4 in 12 months), chronic effusion >3 months, suspected hearing loss.

Pharyngitis / Tonsillitis

- **Most viral** (adenovirus, rhinovirus); bacterial = Group A strep.
- **Centor criteria (children):** fever, tonsillar exudates, tender cervical nodes, absence of cough.
- **Office Management:**
    - Rapid strep test or throat culture if Centor ≥2.
    - GAS confirmed → penicillin V or amoxicillin × 10 days.
    - Supportive care if viral.
- **ED Referral:** airway compromise (stridor, drooling, trismus → consider peritonsillar or retropharyngeal abscess).
- **Specialist Referral:** ENT for recurrent strep tonsillitis, sleep-disordered breathing, suspected abscess.

Bronchiolitis

- **Etiology:** RSV most common; affects infants <2 yrs.
- **Presentation:** rhinorrhea, cough, wheeze, tachypnea, feeding difficulty.
- **Office Management:**
  - Supportive only: hydration, nasal suction, oxygen if hypoxemic.
  - No role for antibiotics, steroids, bronchodilators in typical cases.
- **ED Referral:** severe respiratory distress, O2 sat <90%, apnea, poor oral intake, dehydration.
- **Specialist Referral:** pediatric respirology if recurrent/severe cases, underlying lung/heart disease.

Community-Acquired Pneumonia (CAP)

- **Presentation:** fever, tachypnea, cough, chest pain, crackles, decreased breath sounds.
- **Office Management:**
  - CXR not required unless atypical or severe.
  - Outpatient:
    - <5 yrs: amoxicillin.
    - ≥5 yrs: amoxicillin or macrolide (atypical).
- **ED Referral:** hypoxemia, dehydration, sepsis, respiratory distress.

- **Specialist Referral:** recurrent pneumonia, suspected aspiration or immunodeficiency.

Acute Gastroenteritis (AGE)

- **Etiology:** viral (rotavirus, norovirus, adenovirus).
- **Presentation:** vomiting, diarrhea, fever, dehydration.
- **Office Management:**
    - Assess hydration (urine output, tears, mucous membranes, cap refill).
    - Oral rehydration solution (ORS) is first-line.
    - Avoid antimotility agents.
    - Antibiotics only if bacterial suspicion (bloody diarrhea, high fever, outbreak).
- **ED Referral:** severe dehydration, shock, persistent vomiting, altered mental status.
- **Specialist Referral:** pediatric GI if recurrent, chronic diarrhea, failure to thrive.

Other Key Pediatric Infections to Recognize

- **Hand-Foot-Mouth Disease (Coxsackie):** supportive only, good hand hygiene.
- **Varicella (chickenpox):** supportive; acyclovir for immunocompromised or severe.
- **Influenza:** antiviral if high risk or severe.
- **Pertussis:** prolonged cough, paroxysms, post-tussive vomiting → macrolide antibiotics, reportable disease.

Office / Primary Care Approach (General Principles)

- Careful history: onset, fever, feeding, hydration, exposures, vaccination status.
- Focused exam: vitals, hydration, respiratory effort, ENT.
- Supportive management emphasized.
- Judicious antibiotic use – most infections viral.
- Parental education: red flags (respiratory distress, poor oral intake, lethargy, persistent fever).

When to Refer to ED (Urgent – General Triggers)

- Age <2 months with fever.
- Signs of sepsis: poor perfusion, altered mental status, tachycardia.
- Hypoxemia, respiratory distress.
- Severe dehydration or shock.
- Concern for meningitis, encephalitis, abscess.

When to Refer to Specialists (Non-Urgent)

- ENT: recurrent otitis, chronic tonsillitis, hearing/speech delay.
- Respirology: recurrent bronchiolitis, asthma suspicion.
- Immunology: recurrent infections, failure to thrive.
- GI: chronic diarrhea, poor growth.

Long-Term / Prevention

- Routine immunizations (PCV, Hib, MMR, varicella, influenza).
- Breastfeeding reduces risk of otitis, gastroenteritis, lower respiratory infections.
- Hand hygiene, daycare education.
- Avoid unnecessary antibiotics to reduce resistance.

Pocket Box – Common Pediatric Infections Quick Reference

- **AOM:** pain control ± amoxicillin; refer ENT if recurrent.
- **Strep throat:** test if Centor ≥2; treat if positive.
- **Bronchiolitis:** supportive only; admit if hypoxemia or feeding issues.
- **CAP:** amoxicillin; refer ED if severe.

AGE: ORS first-line; refer ED if dehydrated.

56. Pediatric Respiratory Conditions

Introduction

Respiratory illnesses are among the most common presentations in pediatric practice. While most are self-limited viral infections, others require urgent recognition and intervention. Family physicians are often the first to assess children with cough, wheeze, or respiratory distress, making it essential to distinguish benign from life-threatening illness.

Asthma in Children

Presentation

- Recurrent cough, wheeze, shortness of breath, exercise intolerance.
- Symptoms often worse at night or early morning.
- Triggers: viral infections, allergens, exercise, cold air.

Diagnosis

- <6 yrs: clinical diagnosis (no reliable spirometry).
- ≥6 yrs: spirometry with bronchodilator reversibility.
- Rule out alternative diagnoses (foreign body, bronchiolitis, reflux).

Office Management

- **Mild intermittent:** SABA PRN.
- **Persistent asthma:** daily inhaled corticosteroid (ICS); SABA PRN.
- **Moderate-severe:** step up to ICS-LABA or higher-dose ICS.
- Education: inhaler technique, adherence, trigger avoidance.
- Provide **written asthma action plan** to family.

When to Refer to ED (Urgent)

- Severe attack: difficulty speaking, tachypnea, O2 sat <92%, accessory muscle use, silent chest.

When to Refer to Specialists

- Pediatric respirology if poor control despite step-up therapy, frequent exacerbations, suspected alternative diagnosis.

Croup (Viral Laryngotracheobronchitis)

Presentation

- Barking cough, inspiratory stridor, hoarseness, worse at night.
- Usually ages 6 months – 6 years.

Office Management

- Mild (no stridor at rest): supportive, cool air, fluids.
- Moderate-severe: oral dexamethasone (**0.15–0.6 mg/kg**) single dose or oral prednisolone **1 mg/kg** single dose.
- Nebulized epinephrine if stridor at rest, significant distress.

When to Refer to ED (Urgent)

- Stridor at rest not responding to treatment.
- Severe respiratory distress or hypoxia.

When to Refer to Specialists

- ENT: recurrent or atypical croup, suspected anatomical airway issue.

Pertussis (Whooping Cough)

Presentation

- Catarrhal phase: mild URI symptoms.
- Paroxysmal phase: severe coughing fits, inspiratory "whoop," post-tussive vomiting.
- Convalescent phase: gradual improvement over weeks.

Office Management

- Early: macrolide (azithromycin/clarithromycin).
- Supportive: hydration, monitor for apnea in infants.
- Notify public health (reportable disease).
- Chemoprophylaxis for close contacts.

When to Refer to ED (Urgent)

- Infants <6 months (risk of apnea, death).
- Severe paroxysms with cyanosis, hypoxia, pneumonia.

When to Refer to Specialists

- Infectious disease if complicated or immunocompromised.

Wheeze in Infants

Differential

- Bronchiolitis (RSV).
- Asthma/reactive airway disease.
- Viral-induced wheeze.
- Anatomic airway anomaly (tracheomalacia, vascular ring).
- Foreign body aspiration.

Office Management

- Trial of SABA if >12 months and asthma suspected.
- Supportive care if bronchiolitis (suction, hydration, oxygen if low sats).
- Education: natural history, warning signs.

When to Refer to ED (Urgent)

- Moderate-severe respiratory distress (retractions, grunting, O2 sat <90%).
- Suspected foreign body aspiration with unilateral wheeze/stridor.

When to Refer to Specialists

- Pediatric respirology: recurrent wheeze, suspected asthma not responding to therapy.
- ENT/pulmonology: congenital airway anomaly.

Office / Primary Care General Principles for Pediatric Resp

- Assess severity: work of breathing, O2 saturation, feeding, hydration.
- Supportive care first; oxygen if hypoxemic.
- Minimize unnecessary antibiotics.
- Educate caregivers on red flags: increased work of breathing, lethargy, poor feeding, cyanosis.

Long-Term / Prevention

- Encourage influenza and pertussis (Tdap) vaccination.
- Promote smoke-free homes.
- Asthma: action plans, annual review, update inhaler technique.
- Educate families on infection control: hand hygiene, reduce daycare spread.

Pocket Box – Pediatric Resp Quick Reference

- **Asthma:** ICS if persistent; action plan; ED if severe attack.
- **Croup:** dexamethasone or prednisolone; ED if stridor at rest persists.

- **Pertussis:** macrolide; report to public health; ED if <6mo.

Infant wheeze: trial SABA >12mo; ED if distress/hypoxia/FB.

57. Pediatric GI & Nutrition

Introduction

Gastrointestinal and nutrition-related concerns are frequent in pediatric practice, ranging from benign feeding issues to conditions requiring urgent intervention. Family physicians play a key role in early diagnosis, reassurance, parental counselling, and timely referral when red flags are identified.

Infant Colic & Reflux

Colic

- **Definition:** excessive crying ≥3 hrs/day, ≥3 days/week, ≥3 weeks, otherwise healthy infant.
- **Management in Office:**
    - Reassure parents: peaks at 6 weeks, resolves by 3–4 months.
    - Encourage soothing techniques: swaddling, rocking, white noise.
    - Avoid unnecessary formula changes or medications.

Reflux (GER vs GERD)

- **Physiologic reflux:** common, peaks at 4 months, resolves by 12–18 months.
- **GERD (pathologic):** poor weight gain, feeding refusal, hematemesis, apnea, chronic cough.
- **Office Management:**
    - Conservative: smaller frequent feeds, upright positioning after feeding, thickened feeds.
    - Avoid acid suppression unless red flags (poor growth, severe symptoms).
- **ED Referral:** hematemesis, apnea, severe dehydration.
- **Specialist Referral:** pediatric GI if persistent GERD, poor growth, or complications.

Constipation

Presentation

- Infrequent, hard stools, pain with defecation, withholding behavior, encopresis.

Office Management

- Rule out secondary causes (hypothyroidism, Hirschsprung, spinal abnormality).

- First-line: **polyethylene glycol (PEG 3350)**, titrate to daily soft stool.
- Encourage fluids, high-fiber diet, regular toilet sitting.
- Behavioural support, reward system.

ED Referral

- Severe abdominal distension, vomiting, obstruction.

Specialist Referral

- Pediatric GI if refractory to therapy, failure to thrive, red flags (delayed meconium, neurologic signs).

Diarrhea & Dehydration

Acute diarrhea

- Usually viral (rotavirus, norovirus, adenovirus).
- Assess hydration: urine output, mucous membranes, capillary refill, tear production.

Office Management

- Oral rehydration solution (ORS) first-line.

- Continue breastfeeding/formula; avoid juice/sugary drinks.
- Probiotics may shorten duration.
- Antibiotics rarely indicated (consider only if bacterial suspicion: bloody stools, high fever, outbreak).

ED Referral

- Severe dehydration, shock, altered consciousness, intractable vomiting.

Specialist Referral

- Pediatric GI if chronic/recurrent diarrhea, failure to thrive, suspected IBD or celiac.

Celiac Disease (Pediatric Considerations)

Presentation

- Chronic diarrhea, poor growth, abdominal distension, irritability.
- May present with atypical features: anemia, delayed puberty, dental enamel defects.

Investigations

- Anti-tTG IgA (with total IgA).

- If positive → refer to pediatric GI for biopsy confirmation.

Office Management

- Do not start gluten-free diet before diagnostic workup.
- Monitor growth, nutrition, bone health once diagnosed.

Failure to Thrive (FTT)

Definition

- Weight <3rd percentile or crossing >2 major percentiles downward.

Causes

- Inadequate intake (feeding issues, neglect).
- Malabsorption (celiac, cystic fibrosis, chronic diarrhea).
- Increased metabolic demand (CHD, chronic illness).

Office Management

- Detailed feeding history, growth chart review.
- Screen for iron deficiency, celiac, thyroid, chronic illness.

- Provide nutritional counselling, high-calorie foods, frequent meals.

ED Referral

- Severe malnutrition, dehydration, hemodynamic instability.

Specialist Referral

- Pediatric GI/nutrition for persistent FTT.
- Consider social services if neglect suspected.

Office / Primary Care General Approach

- Growth chart review is critical at every visit.
- Detailed feeding and stooling history for GI complaints.
- Provide anticipatory guidance on nutrition (solids at 6 months, avoid juice, healthy toddler diet).
- Reinforce hydration and safe feeding practices.

Long-Term / Prevention

- Promote exclusive breastfeeding to 6 months.
- Encourage family meals, balanced diet, avoid sugary drinks.
- Vitamin D supplementation in infants and children.
- Early recognition of celiac and other chronic GI conditions.
- Support for parents: feeding guidance, reassurance, mental health support.

Pocket Box – Pediatric GI Quick Reference

- **Colic:** reassure; resolves by 3–4 mo.
- **Reflux:** conservative → refer if poor growth.
- **Constipation:** PEG 3350 + dietary measures; refer if red flags.
- **Diarrhea:** ORS first-line; refer ED if dehydration/shock.
- **Celiac:** screen with anti-tTG IgA; confirm with biopsy.

FTT: growth chart + feeding history; refer GI if persistent.

58. Pediatric Dermatology

Introduction

Skin problems are a common reason for pediatric visits in family medicine. Most are benign and self-limited, but some require prompt recognition and treatment to prevent complications. Parents often worry about rashes, so clear counselling and reassurance are key.

Atopic Dermatitis (Eczema)

Presentation

- Chronic, relapsing pruritic rash.
- Infants: cheeks, scalp, extensor surfaces.
- Older children: flexural surfaces (elbows, knees, neck).
- Associated with asthma, allergic rhinitis (atopic triad).

Office Management

- Daily emollients (ointment/cream preferred over lotion).
- Avoid irritants: harsh soaps, fragrances.

- Topical steroids:
  - Mild (hydrocortisone 1%) for face, flexures.
  - Moderate–potent (betamethasone, mometasone) for body flares.
- Antihistamines if severe pruritus interfering with sleep.
- Treat secondary infection (impetiginization) with topical or oral antibiotics.

When to Refer to ED

- Eczema herpeticum (fever, widespread vesicles/pustules).
- Severe secondary infection with systemic illness.

When to Refer to Specialists

- Dermatology: severe/refractory eczema, suspected contact dermatitis.
- Allergy: if multiple food/environmental allergies suspected.

Diaper Dermatitis

Causes

- Irritant (most common).

- Candidal: beefy red rash with satellite lesions.
- Bacterial: perianal streptococcal dermatitis.

Office Management

- Frequent diaper changes, gentle cleansing, air exposure.
- Barrier creams (zinc oxide, petroleum jelly).
- Antifungal cream (nystatin, clotrimazole) if candida suspected.
- Antibiotics if bacterial superinfection.

When to Refer to ED

- Rare — only if severe systemic illness with cellulitis.

When to Refer to Specialists

- Dermatology for recurrent/refractory cases.

Impetigo

Presentation

- Superficial bacterial infection (Staph aureus, GAS).

- Honey-colored crusted lesions, often on face/extremities.
- Highly contagious.

Office Management

- Localized: mupirocin ointment.
- Widespread: oral cephalexin or cloxacillin.
- Counsel on hygiene, avoid sharing towels.

When to Refer to ED

- Signs of systemic illness, rapidly spreading cellulitis.

When to Refer to Specialists

- Recurrent impetigo, MRSA suspicion, unusual presentation.

Viral Exanthems

Common Types

- Measles: fever, cough, coryza, conjunctivitis, Koplik spots, maculopapular rash.
- Varicella: vesicular rash in crops, various stages.

- Roseola: high fever then sudden rash as fever subsides.
- Hand-Foot-Mouth Disease: vesicles on oral mucosa, palms, soles, buttocks.

Office Management

- Mostly supportive: fluids, antipyretics, rest.
- Isolation: varicella, measles (reportable).
- Education for parents: natural course, red flags.

When to Refer to ED

- Measles with pneumonia/encephalitis signs.
- Varicella with complications (encephalitis, sepsis, secondary infection).
- Severe dehydration due to poor oral intake.

When to Refer to Specialists

- Infectious disease for complex or immunocompromised cases.

Poison Ivy / Allergic Contact Dermatitis

Presentation

- Linear vesicular rash on exposed areas after contact.
- Very pruritic, may ooze or crust.

Office Management

- Wash skin and clothes promptly after exposure.
- Topical steroids for mild cases.
- Oral antihistamines for itch.
- Severe widespread cases: oral prednisone 1 mg/kg × 5–7 days.

When to Refer to ED

- Rare: extensive facial/genital swelling, anaphylaxis-like reaction.

When to Refer to Specialists

- Dermatology for recurrent or unclear contact dermatitis.

Office / Primary Care General Principles

- Careful history: onset, distribution, associated systemic symptoms, exposures.
- Exam: morphology, distribution, secondary infection signs.

- Management: supportive care, targeted topical/systemic therapy.
- Educate parents: expected course, avoid overuse of steroids, red flag signs.

Long-Term / Prevention

- Atopic dermatitis: daily moisturizers, avoid triggers.
- Diaper rash: barrier protection, frequent diaper changes.
- Impetigo: good hygiene, cut nails short.
- Viral exanthems: ensure immunizations up to date.
- Poison ivy: teach recognition of plant, protective clothing.

Pocket Box – Pediatric Dermatology Quick Reference

- **Eczema:** emollients + topical steroids for flares; refer ED if eczema herpeticum.
- **Diaper rash:** barrier creams; add antifungal if candida.
- **Impetigo:** mupirocin if mild, oral cephalexin if widespread.

- **Viral exanthems:** supportive care; report measles/varicella.

Poison ivy: topical steroids; oral prednisone if severe/widespread.

59. Pediatric Neurology

Introduction

Neurological presentations in children can be alarming for families and challenging for physicians. While many are benign (e.g., febrile seizures), others require urgent recognition and referral. Family physicians should focus on early detection, parental reassurance, and timely referral when red flags are present.

Febrile Seizures

Definition

- Generalized seizure in a child **6 months–5 years**, associated with fever but without CNS infection or metabolic disturbance.
- **Simple:** generalized, <15 min, once in 24 hrs.
- **Complex:** focal, >15 min, or recurrent within 24 hrs.

Office Management

- Reassure parents: generally benign, no long-term epilepsy risk in simple cases.

- Treat fever with antipyretics (comfort, not prevention of seizures).
- No routine anticonvulsants.

When to Refer to ED

- First seizure (rule out meningitis, intracranial pathology).
- Complex seizure.
- Prolonged seizure (>5 min → give buccal midazolam or rectal diazepam if available).

When to Refer to Specialists

- Pediatric neurology: recurrent, complex seizures, developmental delay, abnormal exam.

Epilepsy

Definition

- ≥2 unprovoked seizures >24 hrs apart, or single seizure with high recurrence risk.

Office Management

- Detailed history (semiology, triggers, family history).

- Baseline labs, EEG, neuroimaging ordered by neurology.
- Avoid driving/biking/swimming unsupervised until cleared.
- Counsel parents: seizure first aid (place child on side, do not restrain, call EMS if >5 min).

When to Refer to ED

- Status epilepticus (>5 min continuous seizure, or recurrent without recovery).
- New seizure with fever → rule out CNS infection.

When to Refer to Specialists

- Pediatric neurology for all confirmed/suspected epilepsy.
- Urgent referral if abnormal neuro exam, developmental regression, or refractory seizures.

Developmental Delay & Autism Spectrum Disorder (ASD)

Developmental Delay

- Delay in one or more domains (motor, language, cognitive, social).
- Screen with ASQ at well-child visits.

Autism Spectrum Disorder

- Features: language delay, poor eye contact, lack of social reciprocity, repetitive behaviours.
- Screen with M-CHAT at 18–24 months.

Office Management

- Early identification and referral = best outcomes.
- Order hearing test, lead screen if indicated.
- Provide family support, educational resources.

When to Refer to Specialists

- Developmental pediatrics, psychology, speech-language pathology, occupational therapy.
- Neurology if regression, seizures, abnormal neuro exam.

Cerebral Palsy (CP)

Definition

- Permanent, non-progressive motor impairment due to early brain injury.

Presentation

- Spasticity, dystonia, poor coordination.
- May have seizures, intellectual disability, feeding problems.

Office Management

- Monitor growth, nutrition, development.
- Vaccinations, anticipatory guidance.
- Support families with community resources.

When to Refer to Specialists

- Pediatric neurology, physiatry, physiotherapy, OT, speech-language therapy.
- Orthopedics for contractures/scoliosis.

Office / Primary Care General Principles

- Take a detailed birth/developmental history.
- Screen for milestones at every well-child visit.
- Educate families about prognosis, red flags, and when to seek urgent care.

- Provide ongoing support and coordination with multidisciplinary teams.

When to Refer to ED (General Triggers)

- First seizure (esp. <1 yr).
- Seizure >5 min (status epilepticus).
- Seizure with fever → rule out meningitis/encephalitis.
- Acute regression of developmental milestones.

Long-Term / Prevention

- Promote early intervention in developmental delay/ASD.
- Vaccination (prevents meningitis/encephalitis that can cause seizures/CP).
- Support families with education and resources.
- Monitor school performance, behaviour, and social skills.

Pocket Box – Pediatric Neuro Quick Reference

- **Febrile seizure:** benign, reassure; ED if first/complex/prolonged.
- **Epilepsy:** ≥2 seizures; always refer to neurology.
- **Developmental delay/ASD:** screen with ASQ, M-CHAT; refer early.

CP: supportive care, refer to multidisciplinary team.

60. Pediatric Musculoskeletal & Injuries

Introduction

Musculoskeletal presentations are common in pediatrics, ranging from benign growth-related pains to serious injuries and developmental disorders. Family physicians must differentiate between self-limited conditions and those needing urgent evaluation or referral.

Developmental Dysplasia of the Hip (DDH)

Presentation & Risk Factors

- Risk: breech presentation, family history, female, oligohydramnios.
- Presentation: asymmetric thigh/gluteal folds, leg length discrepancy, limited abduction.

Office Management

- Screen newborns with Ortolani and Barlow maneuvers.
- After 2–3 months: limited abduction more reliable than Barlow/Ortolani.

- Imaging:
    - Ultrasound if <6 months with risk factors or abnormal exam.
    - X-ray if >6 months.

When to Refer to ED

- Not typically urgent unless acute hip dislocation with pain.

When to Refer to Specialists

- Orthopedics if abnormal exam or imaging.
- All confirmed cases → early referral = best outcomes.

Growing Pains vs Red Flags

Growing Pains

- Bilateral leg pain, evenings/night, normal physical exam, no limp, resolves with massage/analgesia.

Red Flags (require urgent evaluation)

- Persistent, unilateral pain.
- Morning stiffness, systemic symptoms (fever, weight loss, night sweats).
- Limp, limited ROM.
- Bone tenderness or swelling.

Office Management

- Reassure if classic growing pains.
- Educate parents: no activity limitation, normal growth.

When to Refer to ED

- Suspected septic arthritis (febrile, acutely painful joint, unable to bear weight).
- Suspected malignancy (persistent night pain, systemic symptoms, bone swelling).

When to Refer to Specialists

- Orthopedics or rheumatology if red flags or abnormal imaging/labs.

Nursemaid's Elbow (Radial Head Subluxation)

Presentation

- Age 1–4 yrs, sudden refusal to use arm, holding arm pronated and slightly flexed.
- History: traction on arm (pulled by hand/forearm).

Office Management

- Diagnosis is clinical.
- Reduction maneuver:
  - **Supination-flexion:** supinate forearm then flex elbow.
  - **Hyperpronation:** pronate forearm while applying pressure on radial head.
- Success indicated by immediate return of arm use.

When to Refer to ED

- Failure of reduction or severe swelling/deformity (rule out fracture).

When to Refer to Specialists

- Rare; orthopedics if recurrent or atypical presentation.

Fracture Basics in Children

Unique Features

- Growth plates (physeal injuries classified by Salter-Harris).
- Greenstick fractures (incomplete).
- High remodeling potential.

Office Management

- Suspect fracture if pain, swelling, point tenderness, refusal to bear weight.
- Immobilize and arrange X-ray.
- Analgesia: acetaminophen, ibuprofen.
- Splint in office if suspected until imaging confirms.

When to Refer to ED

- Open fractures, neurovascular compromise, compartment syndrome (severe pain, pallor, pulselessness, paresthesia).
- Unstable fractures requiring immediate reduction.

When to Refer to Specialists

- Orthopedics for: displaced, angulated, physeal (Salter-Harris III–V), or intra-articular fractures.
- Recurrent fractures or suspicion of metabolic bone disease.

Office / Primary Care General Principles

- Always assess for trauma history vs non-accidental injury.
- Growth-related pain = benign if classic; investigate if atypical.

- Immobilize and refer when in doubt for fractures.
- Early recognition of DDH improves outcomes dramatically.

Long-Term / Prevention

- Promote injury prevention: helmets, safe play, seatbelts, sports safety.
- Encourage weight-bearing activity and nutrition for bone health.
- Monitor recurrent fractures for underlying pathology.
- Educate families on safe handling of toddlers (avoid pulling by arms).

Pocket Box – Pediatric MSK Quick Reference

- **DDH:** screen with Barlow/Ortolani → US/X-ray → ortho referral.
- **Growing pains:** benign; refer if red flags (unilateral, systemic, limp).
- **Nursemaid's elbow:** reduce in office; ED if failed or atypical.

Fractures: splint, X-ray, analgesia; ED if open/unstable/compartment syndrome.

61. Pediatric Mental Health

Introduction

Mental health concerns in children and adolescents are increasingly common and often present first in primary care. Early recognition, supportive counselling, and timely referral are critical for long-term outcomes. Family physicians provide continuity, family support, and coordination with schools and specialists.

Attention-Deficit/Hyperactivity Disorder (ADHD)

Presentation

- Symptoms before age 12, present in ≥2 settings (home, school).
- Inattention: distractibility, forgetfulness, disorganization.
- Hyperactivity/impulsivity: fidgeting, interrupting, difficulty waiting turn.

Office Management

- Screen with validated tools: SNAP-IV, Vanderbilt.

- Rule out comorbidities (learning disabilities, anxiety, sleep disorders).
- Management:
    - Behavioural interventions: structure, routine, parent training.
    - School supports: IEP, extra time, seating adjustments.
    - Medications: stimulants (methylphenidate, amphetamines); non-stimulants (atomoxetine, guanfacine).
- Regular monitoring of growth, sleep, appetite, mood.

When to Refer to ED

- Rare, unless severe aggression/violence, suicidal ideation, or psychosis.

When to Refer to Specialists

- Child psychiatry or developmental pediatrics if diagnostic uncertainty, severe functional impairment, comorbidities, or poor response to therapy.

Anxiety Disorders

Presentation

- Excessive worry, school refusal, somatic complaints (stomachaches, headaches).
- Separation anxiety in younger children; generalized/social anxiety in older children.

Office Management

- Psychoeducation for child/parents.
- CBT is first-line (school or community-based programs).
- Encourage exposure, gradual return to school/activities.
- Medications: SSRIs (fluoxetine, sertraline) if moderate-severe, or if CBT unavailable/ineffective.

When to Refer to ED

- Severe functional impairment with suicidal thoughts or panic attacks causing syncope/medical instability.

When to Refer to Specialists

- Psychiatry or psychology if severe, refractory, or comorbid depression/ADHD.

Depression in Children & Adolescents

Presentation

- Persistent sadness, irritability, withdrawal, changes in sleep/appetite.
- Decline in school performance, social withdrawal.
- May present with somatic complaints (headache, abdominal pain).

Office Management

- Screen with PHQ-9 (adolescent version) or CES-DC.
- Assess for suicidality at every visit.
- Mild cases: supportive counselling, family therapy, encourage activity and peer support.
- Moderate-severe: CBT, interpersonal therapy; SSRIs (fluoxetine first-line).
- Monitor closely (weekly initially when on SSRIs).

When to Refer to ED

- Suicidal ideation with plan/intent, self-harm, psychosis, severe functional decline.

When to Refer to Specialists

- Psychiatry for moderate-severe depression, suicidality, or treatment resistance.

Eating Disorders (Anorexia, Bulimia, ARFID)

Presentation

- Restrictive eating, excessive exercise, body image distortion.
- Amenorrhea, weight loss, bradycardia, hypotension, electrolyte abnormalities.
- Bulimia: binge-purge cycles, dental erosion, parotid swelling.
- ARFID (avoidant/restrictive food intake disorder): limited food intake without body image disturbance.

Office Management

- Assess weight, BMI, vitals, orthostatic changes.
- Labs: CBC, electrolytes, LFTs, ECG (QT prolongation).
- Family-based therapy (Maudsley approach) is most effective.
- Nutritional rehabilitation and monitoring.
- Medications: SSRIs may help bulimia, anxiety, depression.

When to Refer to ED

- Severe malnutrition, dehydration, electrolyte imbalance, bradycardia, hypotension, arrhythmia, syncope, suicidal ideation.

When to Refer to Specialists

- Multidisciplinary team (pediatrics, psychiatry, dietitian).
- Urgent referral if rapid weight loss or high-risk features.

Office / Primary Care General Principles

- Ask about school, friendships, bullying, family stress.
- Normalize discussion about mental health to reduce stigma.
- Always screen for suicidality in mood disorders.
- Collaborate with parents, schools, and community supports.
- Monitor weight, growth, sleep, school performance regularly.

Long-Term / Prevention

- Encourage resilience: healthy sleep, exercise, social support.
- Promote positive parenting and school engagement.
- Early intervention for behavioural/emotional concerns.

- Support parents and siblings to reduce family stress.

> **Pocket Box – Pediatric Mental Health Quick Reference**
>
> - **ADHD:** SNAP-IV; behaviour + stimulants; refer if refractory.
> - **Anxiety:** CBT first-line; SSRIs if severe.
> - **Depression:** screen with PHQ-9; CBT ± SSRI; ED if suicidality.
>
> **Eating disorders:** monitor vitals/ECG; refer urgent if unstable.

62. Adolescent Medicine

Introduction

Adolescence is a unique developmental stage with rapid physical, psychological, and social changes. Family physicians provide comprehensive care including preventive health, management of common conditions, and guidance on sensitive issues like mental health, sexuality, and substance use. A confidential, youth-friendly approach builds trust and promotes long-term engagement.

Pubertal Development & Variants

Normal Puberty

- Girls: breast development (thelarche) around age 9–11, menarche ~12–13 yrs.
- Boys: testicular enlargement >4 mL at ~11–12 yrs, voice deepening, growth spurt ~13–14 yrs.

Variants

- **Precocious puberty:** girls <8 yrs, boys <9 yrs.

- **Delayed puberty:** no breast by 13 or menarche by 15 (girls); no testicular enlargement by 14 (boys).

Office Management

- Monitor growth, Tanner staging at annual visits.
- Reassure if within normal range.
- Labs (LH, FSH, estradiol/testosterone, TSH, prolactin) if abnormal.

When to Refer to Specialists

- Endocrinology for precocious or delayed puberty, abnormal labs, or suspected pathology.

Menstrual Issues in Teens

Common Problems

- Dysmenorrhea, heavy menstrual bleeding, irregular cycles in first 1–2 years post-menarche.

Office Management

- NSAIDs first-line for dysmenorrhea.
- Combined OCPs or hormonal IUD for heavy or irregular bleeding.

- Rule out bleeding disorders if persistent menorrhagia.

When to Refer to ED

- Severe hemorrhage with hemodynamic instability.

When to Refer to Specialists

- Gynecology if refractory bleeding, PCOS, or suspected bleeding disorder.

Acne Management

Presentation

- Comedones, papules, pustules; may cause scarring, psychosocial distress.

Office Management

- Mild: topical benzoyl peroxide ± topical retinoid.
- Moderate: add topical or oral antibiotics (doxycycline, minocycline).
- Severe/nodulocystic: isotretinoin (requires specialist).
- Counsel on adherence, avoid picking/squeezing.

When to Refer to Specialists

- Dermatology if severe, scarring, or refractory to first-line.

Substance Use Screening & Counselling

Risky Behaviours

- Alcohol, cannabis, vaping, illicit drugs.

Office Management

- Use CRAFFT screening tool.
- Provide brief motivational interviewing.
- Encourage harm reduction, family involvement, community supports.

When to Refer to ED

- Acute intoxication, overdose, suicidal ideation.

When to Refer to Specialists

- Addiction services if persistent/refractory use.
- Psychiatry for comorbid mental illness.

Sexual Health & Contraception

Office Management

- Provide confidential care (see adolescent alone at some point).
- Screen for STIs: chlamydia, gonorrhea, HIV, syphilis, as indicated.
- Counsel on consent, relationships, contraception.
- Contraception:
    - OCPs, POPs, patches, vaginal rings.
    - LARC (IUDs, implants) recommended first-line.
    - Emphasize condoms for STI prevention.

When to Refer to ED

- Sexual assault: urgent referral for forensic exam, prophylaxis (STIs, HIV, pregnancy).

When to Refer to Specialists

- Gynecology for complex contraception needs, abnormal pelvic exam.
- Infectious disease if complicated STI or HIV.

Office / Primary Care General Principles

- Always assess **HEADSS**: Home, Education, Activities, Drugs, Sexuality, Suicide/Mental Health.
- Provide confidential, nonjudgmental care.
- Screen for mental health, substance use, sexual health at every visit.
- Build rapport to support transition into adulthood.

Long-Term / Prevention

- Promote healthy lifestyle: exercise, nutrition, adequate sleep.
- Encourage positive body image, resilience, stress management.
- Preventive care: immunizations (HPV, meningococcal, influenza, Tdap booster).
- Safe driving and injury prevention counselling.
- Support career/education planning.

Pocket Box – Adolescent Medicine Quick Reference

- **Puberty:** monitor Tanner staging; refer if precocious/delayed.
- **Menstrual issues:** NSAIDs → OCPs/IUD; refer if refractory/bleeding disorder.
- **Acne:** topical retinoid/benzoyl peroxide → oral antibiotics → derm if severe.
- **Substance use:** CRAFFT tool + motivational interviewing; ED if overdose.

Sexual health: confidential STI screen + contraception; ED if sexual assault.

Section 9: Geriatric Medicine

63. Dementia, Delirium, Depression in the Elderly

Dementia

Definition: Chronic, progressive decline in cognition and function, interfering with independence.

Causes:

- Alzheimer's disease (most common).
- Vascular dementia.
- Lewy body dementia.
- Frontotemporal dementia.

Initial Office Work-Up:

- Cognitive testing: **MoCA** (preferred), MMSE.
- Bloodwork: CBC, electrolytes, renal/liver, TSH, B12, glucose.
- Screen for depression (rule out pseudodementia).
- CT/MRI if atypical, rapid progression, or focal neuro findings.

Primary Care Management:

- Non-drug: caregiver education/support, safety planning (driving, home).

- Drug: cholinesterase inhibitors (donepezil, rivastigmine, galantamine); memantine for moderate–severe dementia.

When to Refer to ED (Urgent):

- Sudden aggression, danger to self/others.
- Acute deterioration in cognition or function.

When to Refer to Specialists (Non-Urgent):

- Neurology/geriatrics/psychiatry if diagnosis uncertain, young-onset, or refractory behavioural symptoms.

Delirium

Definition: Acute, fluctuating disturbance of attention and cognition due to underlying medical cause.

Causes (DELIRIUM mnemonic):

- **D**rugs (anticholinergics, opioids, benzos).
- **E**lectrolyte imbalance, dehydration.
- **L**ack of drugs (withdrawal).
- **I**nfection (UTI, pneumonia).

- **R**educed sensory input (vision/hearing loss).
- **I**ntracranial (stroke, bleed).
- **U**rinary/fecal retention.
- **M**etabolic (thyroid, hypoglycemia, hepatic/renal).

Initial Office Work-Up:

- History from family (acute onset, fluctuation).
- Vitals, hydration, full exam.
- Labs: CBC, electrolytes, renal/liver, glucose, TSH, urinalysis.
- Consider head CT if no clear cause or neuro signs.

Primary Care Management:

- Identify and treat underlying cause.
- Supportive care: orientation cues, mobility, hydration, sensory aids.
- Avoid restraints and sedatives unless severe agitation risks safety.

When to Refer to ED (Urgent):

- **All cases** of new delirium for urgent evaluation.

Depression in the Elderly

Definition: Persistent low mood, anhedonia, or functional decline ≥2 weeks. May mimic dementia ("pseudodementia").

Causes / Risk Factors:

- Chronic illness, bereavement, social isolation, polypharmacy.
- Medications: beta-blockers, benzos, corticosteroids.

Initial Office Work-Up:

- Screen with Geriatric Depression Scale (GDS).
- Rule out hypothyroidism, B12 deficiency, anemia.
- Assess suicidality at every visit.

Primary Care Management:

- Mild: counselling, social engagement, physical activity.
- Moderate-severe: CBT, interpersonal therapy, SSRIs (sertraline, citalopram preferred).
- Avoid TCAs (anticholinergic, cardiac risk).

When to Refer to ED (Urgent):

- Suicidal ideation or attempt.
- Severe functional decline with inability to care for self.

When to Refer to Specialists (Non-Urgent):

- Psychiatry for resistant depression, psychosis, or diagnostic uncertainty.

Pocket Box – Office Cognitive & Mood Disorders Quick Reference

- **Dementia:** gradual/progressive → MoCA/MMSE → cholinesterase inhibitors ± memantine → refer if atypical/young/refractory.
- **Delirium:** acute/fluctuating → identify cause → always ED.

Depression: screen with GDS → SSRIs first-line → ED if suicidal.

64. Frailty & Falls Assessment

Frailty

Definition: A clinical state of increased vulnerability due to decline across multiple physiological systems.

Causes / Risk Factors:

- Age >75, chronic diseases, malnutrition, polypharmacy, cognitive decline, social isolation.

Initial Office Work-Up:

- Screening: Clinical Frailty Scale (CFS), Edmonton Frail Scale.
- Functional assessment: ADLs, IADLs.
- Review weight loss, gait speed, grip strength, fatigue.
- Labs: CBC, electrolytes, renal/liver, TSH, vitamin D, B12 if unexplained decline.

Primary Care Management:

- Encourage strength/balance exercise programs.

- Nutrition: adequate protein, vitamin D/calcium supplementation.
- Review & optimize chronic disease management.
- Advance care planning (ACP) discussions.

When to Refer to ED (Urgent):

- Acute decline with injury, dehydration, or infection.
- Syncope or collapse with hemodynamic instability.

When to Refer to Specialists (Non-Urgent):

- Geriatrics for comprehensive assessment in moderate–severe frailty.
- Allied health: PT/OT, dietitian, social work for functional support.

Falls

Definition: Involuntary event leading to rest on ground or lower level, not due to overwhelming external force.

Causes / Risk Factors:

- Intrinsic: frailty, balance/gait disorders, vision/hearing loss, neuropathy, orthostatic hypotension, dementia.

- Extrinsic: environmental hazards (poor lighting, loose rugs), inappropriate footwear, mobility aids.
- Medications: sedatives, antihypertensives, anticholinergics, polypharmacy.

Initial Office Work-Up:

- History: circumstances of fall, frequency, prodromal symptoms (dizziness, syncope).
- Exam: vitals with orthostatics, gait/balance (Timed Up and Go test), neuro, cardiac, vision.
- Medications: review and deprescribe high-risk drugs.
- Labs (if indicated): CBC, electrolytes, glucose, TSH, B12.

Primary Care Management:

- Fall prevention counselling: safe footwear, walking aids.
- Exercise: balance/strength training, community fall prevention programs.
- Environmental modifications: home safety assessment, grab bars, improved lighting.
- Optimize vision/hearing.
- Vitamin D ± calcium supplementation.

When to Refer to ED (Urgent):

- Fall with head injury, suspected fracture, or major trauma.
- Syncope-related fall with concerning features (arrhythmia, stroke, seizure).

When to Refer to Specialists (Non-Urgent):

- Geriatrics for recurrent unexplained falls.
- PT/OT for gait and balance training, home safety evaluation.
- Cardiology/neurology if underlying arrhythmia, seizure, or neuro cause suspected.

Pocket Box – Frailty & Falls Quick Reference

- **Frailty:** screen with CFS/Edmonton scale → exercise + nutrition → ACP.
- **Falls:** history, orthostatics, gait test, med review → exercise + home safety + vit D.
- **Refer ED:** acute trauma, syncope with red flags.

Refer Specialists: geriatrics (frailty, recurrent falls), PT/OT (mobility), cardio/neuro if indicated.

65. Polypharmacy Management

Definition

- **Polypharmacy:** use of ≥5 medications daily.
- **Problematic polypharmacy:** use of multiple drugs with more harm than benefit.

Causes / Risk Factors

- Multiple chronic diseases (diabetes, hypertension, heart failure, COPD).
- Fragmented care (multiple prescribers).
- Age-related changes in pharmacokinetics/pharmacodynamics.
- Poor medication reconciliation at transitions of care.

Risks / Complications

- Adverse drug reactions (falls, delirium, bleeding, renal/hepatic toxicity).

- Drug–drug interactions (warfarin, DOACs, digoxin, SSRIs).
- Medication non-adherence (complex regimens, cost).
- Functional decline, hospitalizations, mortality.

Initial Office Work-Up

- Comprehensive medication review (prescribed, OTC, supplements).
- Check indication, dose, duplication, duration.
- Review for high-risk meds in elderly: anticholinergics, benzos, opioids, antipsychotics.
- Apply tools: Beers Criteria, STOPP/START criteria.
- Assess adherence, patient understanding, ability to self-manage.

Primary Care Management

- **Deprescribing:** taper/stop unnecessary meds (e.g., benzos, PPIs, anticholinergics).
- **Simplify regimens:** once-daily dosing, blister packs, pharmacy synchronization.

- **Shared decision-making:** involve patient/caregiver in medication goals.
- **Regular review:** at least annually, or every 6 months in frail patients.
- **Non-drug alternatives:** lifestyle interventions where appropriate.

When to Refer to ED (Urgent)

- Suspected serious adverse drug reaction (GI bleed, arrhythmia, severe hypoglycemia).
- Acute delirium, fall, or syncope likely medication-related.

When to Refer to Specialists (Non-Urgent)

- Clinical pharmacy/geriatrics: complex polypharmacy, multiple prescribers, high frailty burden.
- Psychiatry: psychotropic polypharmacy or treatment-resistant mental illness.

Pocket Box – Polypharmacy Quick Reference

- **Review all meds** (Rx + OTC + supplements) regularly.
- **Deprescribe high-risk drugs** (benzos, anticholinergics, PPIs, opioids).
- **Use tools** (Beers, STOPP/START).
- **ED:** ADR, fall, delirium, bleed.

Specialists: geriatrics/pharmacy for complex cases.

66. Palliative and End-of-Life Care

Definition

- **Palliative care:** holistic approach to improve quality of life for patients with life-limiting illness.
- **End-of-life care:** last weeks–months of life, focusing on comfort, dignity, and support for family.

Common Indications

- Advanced cancer.
- End-stage organ failure (CHF, COPD, CKD, cirrhosis).
- Advanced dementia or neurodegenerative disease.

Core Principles

- Patient- and family-centred care.
- Symptom control (pain, dyspnea, nausea, anxiety).

- Communication: clear, compassionate, ongoing discussions about goals of care.
- Advance care planning (ACP) and medical orders for scope of treatment (MOST/MOLST).

Initial Office Work-Up

- Assess prognosis, illness trajectory.
- Review medications: discontinue non-essential drugs (statins, tight glycemic control).
- Evaluate symptoms with standardized tools (ESAS-r).
- Screen for psychosocial, spiritual, and caregiver needs.

Primary Care Management

- **Pain:** stepwise approach (acetaminophen → opioids; adjuvants for neuropathic pain).
- **Dyspnea:** opioids, oxygen if hypoxemic, non-drug measures (fan, positioning).
- **Nausea/vomiting:** dopamine antagonists (metoclopramide), antihistamines, serotonin antagonists.

- **Anxiety/agitation:** reassurance, counselling, benzodiazepines if needed.
- **Constipation:** always prophylax with opioids.
- **Goals of care:** clarify patient's wishes, document resuscitation status (DNR/MOST forms).
- Coordinate with home care, nursing support, hospice where available.

When to Refer to ED (Urgent)

- Severe uncontrolled symptoms (pain crisis, respiratory distress).
- Acute catastrophic event (massive bleed, seizure, fracture) if consistent with patient wishes.
- Only if aligned with patient/family's goals of care (otherwise manage at home/hospice).

When to Refer to Specialists (Non-Urgent)

- Palliative care team: complex symptom management, family conflict, or psychosocial needs.

- Psychiatry/psychology: existential distress, refractory depression/anxiety.
- Spiritual care/social work: holistic support for patient and caregivers.

Pocket Box – Palliative & End-of-Life Care Quick Reference

- **Goals:** comfort, dignity, family support.
- **Management:** pain (opioids), dyspnea (opioids/oxygen), nausea (metoclopramide), constipation prophylaxis.
- **Deprescribe:** non-essential meds (statins, tight DM control).
- **Refer ED:** severe symptom crisis *only if aligned with goals*.

Refer Specialists: palliative team for complex cases.

Section 11: Dermatology

72. Eczema, Psoriasis, Urticaria

Eczema (Atopic Dermatitis)

Definition: Chronic relapsing inflammatory skin condition with pruritus and eczematous lesions.

Presentation:

- Infants: cheeks, scalp, extensor surfaces.
- Children: flexural surfaces (elbows, knees, neck).
- Adults: hands, flexural areas, chronic lichenification.
- Associated with asthma, allergic rhinitis.

Initial Office Work-Up:

- Clinical diagnosis (no routine labs needed).
- Rule out secondary infection if exudate, crusting.

Primary Care Management:

- Daily emollients (ointment/cream preferred).
- Avoid triggers (soaps, fragrances, wool).
- Topical steroids:
    - Low-potency (hydrocortisone) for face/flexures.
    - Medium/high-potency for body flares.
- Oral antihistamines if severe pruritus (esp. for sleep).
- Treat infection: topical/oral antibiotics if impetiginized.

When to Refer to Specialists:

- Dermatology if severe/refractory, unclear diagnosis, or widespread disease.
- Allergy if multiple suspected environmental/food triggers.

Psoriasis

Definition: Chronic autoimmune skin disease with erythematous plaques and silvery scale.

Presentation:

- Plaque psoriasis (elbows, knees, scalp, sacrum).
- Nail pitting, onycholysis.

- May be associated with psoriatic arthritis.

Initial Office Work-Up:

- Clinical diagnosis (biopsy rarely needed).
- Screen for arthritis (joint pain, stiffness, dactylitis).

Primary Care Management:

- Mild–moderate:
    - Topical corticosteroids.
    - Vitamin D analogues (calcipotriol).
    - Coal tar, phototherapy (if available).
- Severe: systemic agents (methotrexate, biologics) → specialist referral.
- Counsel on triggers: infections, stress, alcohol, meds (β-blockers, lithium).

When to Refer to Specialists:

- Dermatology if moderate–severe, >10% BSA, or psoriatic arthritis.
- Rheumatology for suspected psoriatic arthritis.

Urticaria (Hives)

Definition: Transient, pruritic, raised wheals due to mast cell histamine release.

Causes:

- Acute: infections, foods, medications, insect stings.
- Chronic (>6 weeks): autoimmune, idiopathic, thyroid disease.

Presentation:

- Raised, red, itchy wheals that last <24 hrs, may recur.
- Angioedema may accompany.

Initial Office Work-Up:

- Acute: clinical diagnosis, no labs needed.
- Chronic: consider CBC, TSH, ESR/CRP, autoimmune screen if persistent.

Primary Care Management:

- First-line: non-sedating antihistamines (cetirizine, loratadine, fexofenadine).
- Increase dose up to 4× standard if resistant.
- Avoid triggers where possible.

- Short course oral steroids for severe acute cases.

When to Refer to ED (Urgent):

- Urticaria with airway involvement, angioedema, or anaphylaxis.

When to Refer to Specialists:

- Allergy/dermatology if chronic urticaria >6 weeks, refractory to antihistamines.

Pocket Box – Eczema, Psoriasis, Urticaria Quick Reference

- **Eczema:** emollients + topical steroids → refer if severe/refractory.
- **Psoriasis:** plaques + silvery scales → topical steroids/vit D → derm if >10% BSA or arthritis.

Urticaria: antihistamines → ED if airway/angioedema → refer if chronic >6 weeks.

73. Skin Infections (Bacterial, Fungal, Viral)

Bacterial Skin Infections

Common Types:

- **Impetigo:** honey-crusted lesions, usually face/limbs (Strep, Staph).
- **Cellulitis:** erythema, warmth, tenderness, poorly demarcated.
- **Erysipelas:** sharply demarcated erythematous rash, often with fever.
- **Abscess:** localized, fluctuant swelling with pus.

Initial Office Work-Up:

- Clinical diagnosis in most cases.
- CBC, blood cultures if systemic illness.
- Wound swab/aspiration if abscess or recurrent infection.

Primary Care Management:

- Impetigo: topical mupirocin; oral cephalexin if widespread.
- Cellulitis/erysipelas: oral cephalexin or cloxacillin; IV antibiotics if severe/systemic.

- Abscess: incision & drainage ± antibiotics if systemic signs.

When to Refer to ED (Urgent):

- Rapidly spreading cellulitis, systemic toxicity.
- Necrotizing fasciitis suspicion (severe pain out of proportion, bullae, crepitus).

When to Refer to Specialists:

- Dermatology/infectious disease for recurrent, resistant, or atypical infections.

Fungal Skin Infections (Dermatophytes, Candida)

Common Types:

- **Tinea corporis ("ringworm"):** annular, scaly lesion with central clearing.
- **Tinea pedis (athlete's foot).**
- **Tinea capitis:** patchy alopecia, scaling, children.
- **Candidiasis:** intertriginous red rash with satellite lesions.

Initial Office Work-Up:

- Clinical diagnosis usually.
- KOH prep or fungal culture if uncertain.

Primary Care Management:

- Topical antifungals (clotrimazole, terbinafine) for most.
- Oral antifungals (terbinafine, itraconazole, fluconazole) for scalp, nails, extensive disease.
- Keep skin dry, avoid occlusive clothing.

When to Refer to Specialists:

- Dermatology for refractory or recurrent tinea, nail involvement, immunocompromised patients.

Viral Skin Infections

Common Types:

- **Herpes simplex:** grouped vesicles on erythematous base, recurrent.
- **Varicella (chickenpox):** vesicles in different stages, generalized.
- **Herpes zoster (shingles):** dermatomal painful vesicular eruption.

- **Molluscum contagiosum:** umbilicated papules, children/immunocompromised.
- **Warts (HPV):** verrucous papules/plaques.

Initial Office Work-Up:

- Clinical diagnosis in most.
- PCR/viral swabs if diagnosis uncertain.

Primary Care Management:

- HSV: oral acyclovir/valacyclovir.
- Varicella: supportive; antivirals if immunocompromised or high-risk.
- Zoster: oral acyclovir/valacyclovir/famciclovir within 72 hrs of onset.
- Molluscum: self-limited, can use cryotherapy/curettage if bothersome.
- Warts: salicylic acid, cryotherapy; many resolve spontaneously.

When to Refer to ED (Urgent):

- Disseminated HSV/VZV, immunocompromised with systemic illness.
- Zoster ophthalmicus (trigeminal involvement → risk of blindness).

When to Refer to Specialists:

- Dermatology/infectious disease for refractory warts, molluscum in immunocompromised, or recurrent zoster.

> ### Pocket Box – Skin Infections Quick Reference
>
> - **Bacterial:** impetigo → mupirocin; cellulitis → cephalexin; ED if nec fasc.
> - **Fungal:** topical clotrimazole/terbinafine; oral for scalp/nail/widespread.
> - **Viral:** HSV/zoster → acyclovir; molluscum/warts often self-limited.
>
> **Refer ED:** spreading cellulitis, nec fasc, zoster ophthalmicus.

74. Skin Cancers (BCC, SCC, Melanoma)

Basal Cell Carcinoma (BCC)

Definition: Most common skin cancer; locally invasive but rarely metastasizes.

Presentation:

- Pearly papule or nodule with telangiectasia.
- May ulcerate ("rodent ulcer").
- Sun-exposed areas (face, neck, scalp).

Initial Office Work-Up:

- Clinical suspicion.
- Dermoscopy helpful.
- Biopsy (shave/punch) for confirmation.

Primary Care Management:

- Small, low-risk lesions: refer for excision, curettage, or cryotherapy.
- Encourage sun protection, patient education.

When to Refer to Specialists:

- Dermatology/plastic surgery for large, recurrent, or cosmetically sensitive lesions.

Squamous Cell Carcinoma (SCC)

Definition: Malignant proliferation of keratinocytes; can metastasize if high risk.

Presentation:

- Scaly, erythematous plaque or nodule.
- May ulcerate or bleed.
- Arises from actinic keratoses or chronic wounds.
- Common on sun-exposed areas (ears, lips, hands).

Initial Office Work-Up:

- Biopsy for histology.
- Lymph node exam.

Primary Care Management:

- Refer for surgical excision (wide local excision or Mohs).
- Cryotherapy for actinic keratoses.
- Counsel on sun safety.

When to Refer to Specialists:

- Dermatology/oncology for invasive SCC, perineural involvement, or metastasis.

Melanoma

Definition: Malignant tumor of melanocytes; high risk of metastasis and death.

Presentation:

- **ABCDE rule:** Asymmetry, Border irregular, Color variation, Diameter >6 mm, Evolving lesion.
- Subtypes: superficial spreading, nodular, lentigo maligna, acral lentiginous.
- May occur on non–sun-exposed skin, palms, soles, nails.

Initial Office Work-Up:

- Dermoscopy if trained.
- Excisional biopsy with narrow margins (do not shave).
- Staging with Breslow depth.

Primary Care Management:

- Identify suspicious lesions → urgent referral for excision.

- Educate patients on skin self-exam, UV protection.

When to Refer to ED (Urgent):

- Rare, unless bleeding/rapidly ulcerated lesion with systemic compromise.

When to Refer to Specialists:

- Dermatology/oncology for all confirmed melanomas.
- Surgical oncology if high-risk or advanced disease.

Pocket Box – Skin Cancers Quick Reference

- **BCC:** pearly papule, telangiectasia → biopsy → excision/derm referral.
- **SCC:** scaly plaque/nodule, may ulcerate → biopsy → excision.
- **Melanoma:** ABCDE features → excisional biopsy → urgent derm/onc referral.

Sun safety: SPF, protective clothing, avoid tanning beds.

75. Acne & Rosacea

Acne Vulgaris

Definition: Chronic inflammatory disorder of pilosebaceous units.

Presentation:

- **Lesions:** comedones (open = blackheads, closed = whiteheads), papules, pustules, nodules, cysts.
- Common on face, chest, back.
- May cause scarring, psychosocial distress.

Initial Office Work-Up:

- Clinical diagnosis.
- Consider PCOS work-up if irregular menses, hirsutism.

Primary Care Management:

- **Mild acne:**
    - Topical retinoid (adapalene, tretinoin).
    - Benzoyl peroxide (reduces resistance when used with antibiotics).
- **Moderate acne:**

- - Add topical antibiotic (clindamycin) or oral antibiotic (doxycycline, minocycline).
- **Severe acne:**
  - Oral isotretinoin (specialist only, monitor LFTs, lipids, pregnancy prevention).
- **Adjuncts:** gentle cleansing, non-comedogenic skin products, avoid picking.

When to Refer to Specialists:

- Dermatology if severe, scarring, refractory to ≥3 months of standard therapy, or isotretinoin needed.

Rosacea

Definition: Chronic inflammatory skin condition affecting central face.

Subtypes:

- Erythematotelangiectatic (flushing, redness).
- Papulopustular (acne-like lesions without comedones).
- Phymatous (thickened skin, rhinophyma).
- Ocular rosacea (dry, irritated eyes).

Presentation:

- Flushing, persistent central facial erythema.
- Telangiectasia, papules, pustules.
- Worsened by heat, alcohol, spicy foods, sun exposure.

Initial Office Work-Up:

- Clinical diagnosis.
- Rule out acne vulgaris if comedones present (not rosacea).

Primary Care Management:

- Trigger avoidance (sun, alcohol, spicy food, hot drinks).
- Topical metronidazole, azelaic acid, or ivermectin cream.
- Oral tetracyclines (doxycycline, minocycline) for moderate–severe.
- Ocular rosacea: artificial tears, oral tetracyclines if needed.

When to Refer to Specialists:

- Dermatology for refractory or phymatous disease.
- Ophthalmology for ocular rosacea with vision changes.

Pocket Box – Acne & Rosacea Quick Reference

- **Acne:** comedones + papules/pustules → topical retinoid/benzoyl peroxide → add antibiotics if moderate → derm referral if severe.

Rosacea: central face, flushing, no comedones → avoid triggers → topical metronidazole/ivermectin → oral doxycycline if severe.

76. Alopecia

Definition

Loss of hair from scalp or body, classified as **non-scarring (potentially reversible)** or **scarring (permanent, follicle destruction)**.

Non-Scarring Alopecia

Common Types:

- **Androgenetic alopecia (male/female pattern):** gradual thinning at vertex/temples in men; diffuse crown thinning in women.
- **Alopecia areata:** autoimmune, well-demarcated round patches of hair loss; may see exclamation point hairs.
- **Telogen effluvium:** diffuse shedding after stress, illness, childbirth, meds.
- **Trichotillomania:** patchy loss, irregular borders, broken hairs.

Initial Office Work-Up:

- History: timing, triggers, family history, systemic illness.

- Exam: pattern of hair loss, scalp condition.
- Labs if indicated: TSH, ferritin, CBC, vitamin D.

Primary Care Management:

- **Androgenetic:** topical minoxidil; finasteride (men only).
- **Alopecia areata:** topical/intralesional corticosteroids; refer derm if extensive.
- **Telogen effluvium:** reassurance, treat underlying cause; usually self-limited.
- **Trichotillomania:** counselling, behavioural therapy.

When to Refer to Specialists:

- Dermatology if severe alopecia areata, scarring alopecia, or uncertain diagnosis.
- Psychiatry/psychology for trichotillomania.

Scarring Alopecia

Causes:

- Discoid lupus erythematosus.
- Lichen planopilaris.
- Folliculitis decalvans.

Presentation:

- Patchy hair loss with erythema, scaling, pustules, or scarring.
- Follicular openings lost (shiny scalp).

Initial Office Work-Up:

- Clinical exam.
- Scalp biopsy if diagnosis uncertain.

Primary Care Management:

- Early referral to dermatology is essential.
- Supportive scalp care, avoid irritants.

When to Refer to Specialists:

- Dermatology for all suspected scarring alopecia → risk of permanent loss.

Pocket Box – Alopecia Quick Reference

- **Androgenetic:** minoxidil ± finasteride; chronic, progressive.
- **Alopecia areata:** patchy, autoimmune → steroids → derm if extensive.
- **Telogen effluvium:** diffuse shedding, post-stress → self-limited.
- **Trichotillomania:** irregular patches, broken hairs → behavioural therapy.

Scarring alopecia: permanent → urgent derm referral.

This page has been left intentionally blank

Section 12: Mental Health & Psychiatry

77. Depression

Definition

A mood disorder characterized by persistent low mood, anhedonia, and functional impairment lasting ≥2 weeks.

Screening & Diagnosis

- **PHQ-9:** validated screening tool for depression.
    - **Scores:**
        - 0–4: minimal/no depression.
        - 5–9: mild.
        - 10–14: moderate.
        - 15–19: moderately severe.
        - 20–27: severe.
- Must assess functional impact and exclude medical/medication causes (e.g., hypothyroidism, anemia, beta-blockers).
- Always screen for **suicidal ideation** (Q9 of PHQ-9).

Presentation

- Persistent sadness, irritability, loss of interest/pleasure.
- Sleep disturbance, appetite/weight changes.
- Fatigue, poor concentration, guilt, hopelessness.
- Somatic complaints (pain, headaches, GI upset).

Initial Office Work-Up

- History & mental status exam.
- PHQ-9 or other scales (CES-D, HAM-D).
- Labs if indicated: TSH, CBC, B12, glucose, electrolytes.
- Review medications/substance use.

Primary Care Management

- **Mild:** supportive counselling, physical activity, sleep hygiene, problem-solving therapy.
- **Moderate–severe:**
    - First-line: SSRIs (sertraline, citalopram, escitalopram).

    - SNRIs (venlafaxine, duloxetine) or mirtazapine as alternatives.
    - CBT, interpersonal therapy, behavioural activation.
- Monitor response every 2–4 weeks.
- Continue meds for **≥6–12 months** after remission.
- Avoid polypharmacy; switch/augment if poor response.

When to Refer to ED (Urgent)

- Suicidal ideation with plan/intent.
- Suicide attempt or severe self-harm.
- Severe psychomotor retardation or inability to care for self.
- Psychotic depression (hallucinations, delusions).

When to Refer to Specialists (Non-Urgent)

- Psychiatry: treatment-resistant depression, bipolar suspicion, psychotic features, or high suicide risk.
- Psychology: CBT, interpersonal therapy.

- Community mental health resources for psychosocial support.

Pocket Box – Depression Quick Reference

- **Screen:** PHQ-9; always ask about suicidality.
- **Mild:** counselling, exercise, sleep hygiene.
- **Moderate–severe:** SSRIs/SNRIs ± CBT.
- **ED:** suicidality, psychotic depression, inability to care for self.

Specialists: psychiatry for refractory, bipolar suspicion, or complex cases.

78. Anxiety & Panic Disorders

Definition

- **Generalized Anxiety Disorder (GAD):** excessive, uncontrollable worry on most days for ≥6 months, with associated symptoms.
- **Panic Disorder:** recurrent, unexpected panic attacks with persistent concern about future attacks or behavioral changes.

Screening & Diagnosis

- **GAD-7:** validated screening tool.
    - Scores:
        - 0–4: minimal
        - 5–9: mild
        - 10–14: moderate
        - 15–21: severe
- **Panic Disorder:** clinical diagnosis based on panic episodes (sudden surge of intense fear, palpitations, chest pain, SOB, dizziness, fear of dying/losing control).

- Rule out secondary causes: hyperthyroidism, arrhythmias, asthma/COPD, substance use (caffeine, stimulants).

Presentation

- **GAD:** excessive worry, restlessness, irritability, poor concentration, sleep disturbance, muscle tension.
- **Panic Disorder:** sudden episodes of intense fear with autonomic symptoms; may lead to avoidance behaviors and agoraphobia.

Initial Office Work-Up

- History & mental status exam.
- Screening: GAD-7, PHQ-9 (often comorbid depression).
- Rule out organic causes: vitals, thyroid, ECG if cardiac symptoms.

Primary Care Management

- **Non-Pharmacologic:**
  - Psychoeducation and reassurance.

- Cognitive behavioural therapy (CBT) is first-line.
- Relaxation techniques, mindfulness, exercise, sleep hygiene.
- **Pharmacologic:**
  - SSRIs: escitalopram, sertraline, paroxetine.
  - SNRIs: venlafaxine, duloxetine.
  - Buspirone may be considered in GAD.
  - Benzodiazepines: short-term only, for severe acute symptoms or while waiting for SSRIs to take effect (avoid long-term use).

When to Refer to ED (Urgent)

- Severe panic attack mimicking ACS until ruled out (consider ECG, troponins).
- Acute suicidality or self-harm in the context of anxiety/depression.

When to Refer to Specialists (Non-Urgent)

- Psychiatry: treatment-resistant GAD/panic, intolerance to multiple agents, complex comorbidity.
- Psychology: CBT or structured psychotherapy.

Pocket Box – Anxiety & Panic Disorders Quick Reference

- **Screen:** GAD-7; consider PHQ-9 comorbidity.
- **GAD:** worry + ≥3 somatic symptoms ≥6 months.
- **Panic disorder:** recurrent attacks + worry about recurrence.
- **Tx:** CBT + SSRI/SNRI → short-term benzo if severe.

ED: suicidality, rule out ACS in severe panic with chest pain.

79. Bipolar Disorder

Definition

A mood disorder characterized by episodes of **mania/hypomania** and **depression**, with significant impact on functioning.

Diagnostic Features

- **Mania (≥1 week):** elevated/irritable mood, ↑ energy, grandiosity, ↓ need for sleep, pressured speech, racing thoughts, impulsive/risky behavior.
- **Hypomania (≥4 days):** similar but less severe, no marked impairment or hospitalization.
- **Depression:** same as major depressive episode (see 77).
- **Bipolar I:** ≥1 manic episode (± depression).
- **Bipolar II:** ≥1 hypomanic + ≥1 major depressive episode, no full mania.

Screening & Tools

- **Mood Disorder Questionnaire (MDQ):** quick screen for bipolar symptoms.
- Always assess suicide risk (high in both mania and depression).
- Rule out secondary causes (substance use, steroids, thyroid disease).

Presentation in Primary Care

- Patient with recurrent depressive episodes not responding to antidepressants.
- Periods of excessive energy, decreased sleep, impulsivity, risky spending/sexual behavior.
- Family history of bipolar disorder.

Initial Office Work-Up

- Full psychiatric history and MSE.
- Collateral history (often patient insight is limited).
- Labs: TSH, CBC, electrolytes, renal/hepatic function (baseline before mood stabilizers).
- Screen for substance use.

Primary Care Management

- **DO NOT start antidepressants alone** (may trigger mania).
- **Pharmacologic (with psychiatry input):**
    - First-line: mood stabilizers (lithium, valproate, lamotrigine).
    - Atypical antipsychotics: quetiapine, olanzapine, risperidone.
- **Non-Pharmacologic:**
    - Psychoeducation (sleep hygiene, medication adherence, avoid substances).
    - Family support and crisis planning.

When to Refer to ED (Urgent)

- Acute mania with risk of harm to self/others.
- Suicidal ideation/attempt in depressive episode.
- Psychosis with severe impairment.

When to Refer to Specialists (Non-Urgent)

- Psychiatry: all suspected or confirmed bipolar disorder for diagnosis and long-term management.
- Shared care possible after stabilization.

Pocket Box – Bipolar Disorder Quick Reference

- **Dx:** mania ≥1 week, hypomania ≥4 days, alternating with depression.
- **Tx:** mood stabilizers (lithium, valproate, lamotrigine) ± antipsychotics.
- **Avoid:** antidepressant monotherapy.
- **ED:** suicidality, acute mania, psychosis.

Specialists: psychiatry for confirmation & management.

80. Psychosis & Schizophrenia

Definition

Psychosis = loss of contact with reality, presenting with hallucinations, delusions, or disorganized thought/behavior.
Schizophrenia = chronic psychotic disorder lasting ≥6 months with functional impairment.

Diagnostic Features

- **Positive symptoms:** delusions (paranoid, grandiose), hallucinations (auditory > visual), disorganized speech, disorganized/catatonic behavior.
- **Negative symptoms:** flat affect, anhedonia, social withdrawal, poverty of speech.
- **Cognitive symptoms:** impaired attention, working memory, executive function.
- **Schizophrenia criteria:** ≥2 core symptoms (one must be hallucinations, delusions, or disorganized speech)

lasting ≥1 month, with continuous disturbance ≥6 months.

Presentation in Primary Care

- First-episode psychosis (young adults, 15–30 yrs).
- Family brings patient with bizarre behavior, paranoia, withdrawal, or deteriorating function.
- Substance-induced psychosis must be ruled out (cannabis, stimulants, alcohol withdrawal).

Initial Office Work-Up

- Full psychiatric history & mental status exam.
- Collateral history from family (insight often poor).
- Physical exam + vitals.
- Labs: CBC, electrolytes, LFTs, TSH, glucose, B12, HIV/syphilis (if concern).
- Urine toxicology to exclude substance-induced psychosis.
- Consider brain imaging if atypical presentation or neuro findings.

Primary Care Management

- **Acute stabilization:**
    - Ensure safety for patient and others.
    - Antipsychotics: risperidone, olanzapine, quetiapine, haloperidol.
- **Non-Pharmacologic:**
    - Psychoeducation for patient/family.
    - Supportive care: sleep, nutrition, stress reduction.
- Avoid benzodiazepines unless severe agitation.

When to Refer to ED (Urgent)

- First episode psychosis.
- Risk of harm to self or others.
- Severe agitation, aggression, or inability to care for self.
- Suspected organic cause (delirium, encephalitis).

When to Refer to Specialists (Non-Urgent)

- Psychiatry: all cases of confirmed psychotic disorder for long-term management.
- Early psychosis intervention programs if available.
- Community mental health for psychosocial rehabilitation.

Pocket Box – Psychosis & Schizophrenia Quick Reference

- **Dx:** hallucinations, delusions, disorganized thought/behavior.
- **Work-up:** exclude substance/medical causes (tox screen, labs, TSH, B12).
- **Tx:** antipsychotics (risperidone, olanzapine, quetiapine, haloperidol) – with psychiatry input
- **ED:** first-episode, risk to self/others, agitation, organic suspicion.

Specialists: psychiatry for ongoing management.

81. Suicide Risk Assessment

Definition

Systematic evaluation of a patient's risk of self-harm or suicide, integrating history, mental state, and protective/risk factors.

When to Assess

- Any patient with depression, anxiety, psychosis, bipolar disorder, or substance use.
- When presenting with hopelessness, suicidal ideation, self-harm behavior.
- After major psychosocial stressors (loss, trauma, medical diagnosis).

Assessment Framework

1. Direct Inquiry

- Ask clearly and empathetically:
    - "Have you had thoughts of hurting yourself or ending your life?"
    - "Do you have a plan?"

- "Do you have access to means (medications, firearms, rope)?"
- "Have you ever attempted suicide before?"

2. Suicide Risk Factors

- Psychiatric illness: depression, bipolar, psychosis, substance use.
- Past suicide attempt (strongest predictor).
- Family history of suicide.
- Social isolation, unemployment, financial stress.
- Chronic pain or medical illness.

3. Protective Factors

- Strong family/social support.
- Religious/spiritual beliefs.
- Future goals, responsibilities (e.g., children, work).
- Engagement with treatment.

4. Risk Stratification

- **Low risk:** fleeting thoughts, no plan/intent, strong supports.
- **Moderate risk:** frequent thoughts, some intent, limited supports.
- **High risk:** active plan, intent, access to means, history of attempts.

Initial Office Work-Up

- Mental status exam: mood, thought content, judgment, insight.
- Collateral history if possible (family/friends).
- Screen for comorbid depression (PHQ-9), anxiety (GAD-7), substance use.

Primary Care Management

- **Low risk:**
    - Safety planning (remove means, crisis line numbers, close follow-up).
    - Encourage supports and therapy referral.
- **Moderate risk:**
    - Safety plan + involve family/supports.
    - Consider psychiatry referral.
    - Short-term monitoring (weekly or sooner).
- **High risk:**
    - **Do not leave patient alone.**
    - Arrange immediate transfer to ED for psychiatric assessment.
    - May require involuntary admission under mental health act (provincial regulations).

When to Refer to ED (Urgent)

- Active suicidal ideation with plan and intent.
- Access to lethal means.
- Recent suicide attempt.
- Severe psychiatric illness with risk of self-harm.

When to Refer to Specialists (Non-Urgent)

- Psychiatry: ongoing risk, treatment-resistant depression, bipolar disorder, psychosis.
- Counselling/psychology: CBT, DBT, crisis therapy.
- Community mental health teams for case management.

Pocket Box – Suicide Risk Assessment Quick Reference

- **Ask directly**: thoughts, plan, means, prior attempts.
- **Risk factors:** psychiatric illness, past attempts, isolation, medical illness.
- **Protective factors:** family, beliefs, future orientation, treatment engagement.
- **Risk level:**
    - Low → safety plan, follow-up.
    - Moderate → safety plan + psychiatry referral.

High → ED transfer, possible involuntary admission.

Section 13: Infectious Diseases

82. Common Community Infections

Upper Respiratory Tract Infections (URTI)

- **Viral rhinitis/common cold:** supportive (hydration, rest, acetaminophen/NSAIDs, decongestants if needed).
- **Acute bacterial sinusitis:** suspect if ≥10 days persistent, severe onset, or "double sickening."
    - First-line: amoxicillin-clavulanate.
    - Supportive care for viral cases.
- **Pharyngitis:** most viral; strep pharyngitis if Centor/McIsaac score high → throat swab.
    - Tx: penicillin V or amoxicillin x 10 days if Group A strep.

Lower Respiratory Tract Infections

- **Acute bronchitis:** usually viral; antibiotics not indicated unless COPD exacerbation.

- **Community-acquired pneumonia (CAP):**
    - Typical: fever, cough, pleuritic pain, consolidation.
    - Atypical: dry cough, myalgia, headache.
    - Outpatient empiric Tx: amoxicillin OR doxycycline OR azithromycin.
    - CURB-65 score guides admission.

Urinary Tract Infections (UTIs)

Uncomplicated cystitis (non-pregnant women):

- Empiric therapy can be started without culture if clinical features are typical.
- First-line:
    - **Nitrofurantoin 100 mg PO BID x 5 days**
    - **TMP-SMX 1 DS tab PO BID x 3 days** (if local resistance <20%)
    - **Fosfomycin 3 g PO single dose**

Complicated UTIs – Men

- All UTIs in men are considered complicated → **always send urine culture**.
- Empiric treatment (until cultures back):
    - **Ciprofloxacin 500 mg PO BID x 7 days** OR
    - **TMP-SMX DS PO BID x 7 days**
- Consider prostatitis if recurrent/persistent (may need 4–6 weeks of antibiotics).

Pregnant Women

- All symptomatic UTIs require culture & treatment (asymptomatic bacteriuria also needs treatment).
- Safe empiric options (while awaiting culture):
    - **Amoxicillin-clavulanate 500 mg PO TID x 5–7 days**
    - **Cephalexin 500 mg PO QID x 5–7 days**
    - **Fosfomycin 3 g PO single dose**
- **Avoid in pregnancy:**
    - **Fluoroquinolones** (teratogenic, cartilage toxicity).
    - **TMP-SMX** (especially 1st trimester → folate antagonism;

3rd trimester → risk of kernicterus).
- **Nitrofurantoin** should be avoided at term (>38 weeks) due to risk of hemolysis in neonates, but otherwise safe earlier.

Skin & Soft Tissue Infections (SSTIs)

- **Cellulitis:** oral cephalexin or cloxacillin; IV cefazolin if systemic.
- **Impetigo:** topical mupirocin; oral cephalexin if widespread.
- **Abscess:** incision & drainage ± antibiotics if systemic features.

Gastrointestinal Infections

- **Viral gastroenteritis (norovirus, rotavirus):** hydration mainstay.
- **Traveler's diarrhea:** usually bacterial (E. coli).
  - Oral rehydration, loperamide if mild.
  - Consider antibiotics (azithromycin, ciprofloxacin) if severe.

- **C. difficile infection:** risk after antibiotics, PPI.
    - Stop inciting agent.
    - Tx: oral vancomycin or fidaxomicin (metronidazole no longer first-line).

When to Refer to ED (Urgent)

- Severe pneumonia, sepsis, hypotension, hypoxia.
- Pyelonephritis with sepsis features.
- Necrotizing fasciitis suspicion (severe pain, bullae, crepitus).
- Severe dehydration in gastroenteritis.

When to Refer to Specialists

- ID referral for recurrent or resistant infections.
- Urology for recurrent/complicated UTIs.
- Pulmonology if recurrent pneumonia, structural lung disease.

Pocket Box – Common Community Infections Quick Reference

- **URTI:** viral → supportive; strep → penicillin.
- **CAP:** amoxicillin/doxy/azithro outpatient; CURB-65 for admission.
- **UTI:** nitrofurantoin (women); pyelo → fluoroquinolone or IV ceftriaxone.
- **SSTI:** cellulitis → cephalexin; abscess → I&D.
- **GI:** hydration; C. diff → oral vancomycin.

ED: sepsis, severe pneumonia, nec fasc, severe dehydration.

83. STI Screening & Management

Common STIs in Primary Care

- **Chlamydia trachomatis**
- **Neisseria gonorrhoeae**
- **Syphilis**
- **HIV, Hepatitis B & C** (see next for detailed management)
- **HPV (genital warts, cervical dysplasia)**
- **Herpes simplex virus (HSV-1, HSV-2)**
- **Trichomonas vaginalis**

Screening Recommendations (Canada)

- **Routine opportunistic screening:**
    - All sexually active individuals <25 years (chlamydia, gonorrhea).
    - Pregnant women: HIV, syphilis, hepatitis B, chlamydia, gonorrhea.
- **High-risk groups:** MSM (men who have sex with men), sex workers, people with multiple partners, IVDU.

- **Frequency:** annually, or every 3–6 months if high risk.

Initial Office Work-Up

- **History:** sexual partners, practices, contraception, prior STIs, HIV status.
- **Exam:** genital, anal, oral as indicated.
- **Testing:**
    - **NAAT (urine or swab):** chlamydia, gonorrhea.
    - **Serology:** syphilis, HIV, hepatitis B & C.
    - **Wet mount/NAAT:** trichomonas.
    - **Pap smear/HPV testing** as per guidelines.

Empiric Management (while awaiting results, if high suspicion or symptomatic partner exposure)

- **Chlamydia:** doxycycline 100 mg PO BID x 7 days (or azithromycin 1 g PO single dose if adherence concern, but doxy preferred).
- **Gonorrhea:** ceftriaxone 500 mg IM single dose + doxycycline 100 mg PO

BID x 7 days (cover chlamydia co-infection).
- **Syphilis:** benzathine penicillin G 2.4 million units IM single dose (early).
- **HSV (first episode):** acyclovir 400 mg PO TID x 7–10 days or valacyclovir 1 g PO BID x 7–10 days.
- **Trichomonas:** metronidazole 2 g PO single dose or 500 mg PO BID x 7 days.
- **HPV (warts):** cryotherapy, podophyllotoxin, imiquimod cream.

Partner Notification & Public Health

- Mandatory reporting: chlamydia, gonorrhea, syphilis, HIV, hepatitis B.
- Partner notification and treatment required.
- Advise abstinence until treatment completed and partners treated.

When to Refer to ED (Urgent)

- Pelvic inflammatory disease with sepsis signs.
- Disseminated gonococcal infection (arthritis, rash, tenosynovitis).
- Neurosyphilis, ocular syphilis.

- HIV seroconversion illness with severe systemic symptoms.

When to Refer to Specialists (Non-Urgent)

- Infectious disease: HIV management, resistant gonorrhea, syphilis beyond primary stage.
- Gynecology: PID not improving, cervical dysplasia.
- Dermatology: extensive genital warts, refractory HSV.

Pocket Box – STI Quick Reference

- **Screen:** <25 yrs, pregnant women, high-risk groups.
- **Tx (empiric):**
    - Chlamydia → doxycycline 7d.
    - Gonorrhea → ceftriaxone + doxy.
    - Syphilis → benzathine penicillin.
    - HSV → acyclovir/valacyclovir.
    - Trichomonas → metronidazole.
- **Public health:** reportable diseases, partner notification.

ED: PID with sepsis, disseminated GC, neurosyphilis.

84. HIV, Hepatitis B & C

HIV in Primary Care

Who to Screen:

- **Universal once-in-lifetime:** all adults in Canada (opt-out approach).
- **Repeat screening (every 6–12 months):**
    - MSM (men who have sex with men).
    - People who inject drugs (IVDU).
    - Sex workers.
    - Patients with multiple or new sexual partners.
    - Partners of HIV-positive individuals.
    - Pregnant women (universal screening in each pregnancy).

Diagnosis:

- HIV antigen/antibody combo test (4th gen) → confirm with viral load.

Primary Care Role:

- Baseline labs at diagnosis: CBC, renal, liver, CD4, viral load, hepatitis screen, TB testing.

- Vaccinate (influenza, pneumococcal, hepatitis B, HPV if eligible).
- Counsel: safe sex, U=U (undetectable = untransmittable).

Management:

- Refer all to HIV specialists for ART initiation.
- **Primary care ongoing role:** adherence support, chronic disease care, opportunistic infection prevention.
- **PEP:** start within 72 hrs of exposure.
- **PrEP:** tenofovir/emtricitabine daily for high-risk patients.

Hepatitis B (HBV)

Who to Screen:

- All **pregnant women** (universal).
- Individuals from endemic regions (Asia, Africa, Eastern Europe).
- IVDU.
- MSM.
- HIV-positive individuals.
- Household/sexual contacts of HBV carriers.

Diagnosis:

- HBsAg, anti-HBs, anti-HBc (interpretation distinguishes susceptible, immune, chronic, or acute infection).

Primary Care Role:

- **Vaccinate all non-immune individuals.**
- For HBsAg positive patients:
    - Monitor ALT, HBeAg, HBV DNA viral load.
    - HCC surveillance: ultrasound ± AFP q6 months if cirrhosis or high risk.
- Counsel on transmission: sexual, blood, vertical (mother-to-child).

When to Refer:

- Chronic carriers (HBsAg+ >6 months).
- Elevated ALT, high viral load, or cirrhosis.
- Pregnant women with high viral load → hepatology for peripartum management.

Hepatitis C (HCV)

Who to Screen:

- **One-time for all adults in Canada** (regardless of risk).
- High-risk groups for repeated testing:
    - Current or past IVDU.
    - People with HIV.
    - Hemodialysis patients.
    - Received blood transfusion or transplant before 1992.
    - Incarcerated individuals.
- Consider in anyone with unexplained chronic liver disease.

Diagnosis:

- Anti-HCV antibody → confirm with HCV RNA PCR.
- Genotype testing if RNA positive (guides therapy).

Primary Care Role:

- Counsel: harm reduction (needle exchange, avoid sharing razors, safe sex in high-risk groups).
- Vaccinate against hepatitis A & B if non-immune.
- Assess fibrosis (FIB-4, APRI, FibroScan).

Management:

- Refer all RNA-positive patients → direct-acting antivirals (DAAs, cure rates >95%).

- Specialist-led therapy (hepatology/ID) but primary care can support adherence and monitoring.

When to Refer to ED (Urgent)

- Acute liver failure (jaundice, coagulopathy, encephalopathy).
- Severe opportunistic infection in HIV.

When to Refer to Specialists (Non-Urgent)

- HIV: all confirmed cases for ART initiation.
- HBV: chronic infection, cirrhosis, high viral load, pregnancy with HBsAg+.
- HCV: all RNA-positive patients → refer for antiviral therapy.

Pocket Box – Who to Screen

- **HIV:** once in all adults; repeat if MSM, IVDU, sex workers, multiple partners, pregnancy.
- **HBV:** all pregnant women, immigrants from endemic regions, MSM, IVDU, HIV+, household/sexual contacts.

HCV: once in all adults; repeat if IVDU, HIV+, pre-1992 transfusion, dialysis, incarceration.

85. Travel Medicine Essentials

Pre-Travel Assessment in Primary Care

- **Timing:** ideally 4–6 weeks before departure.
- **History:**
  - Destination(s), urban vs rural, season of travel.
  - Duration, purpose (tourism, visiting friends/relatives, work, medical missions).
  - Activities: trekking, camping, sexual exposure, animal contact.
  - Medical history: chronic disease, medications, immunocompromised, pregnancy.
  - Previous immunizations.

Vaccinations

Routine (ensure up to date):

- Tdap, MMR, polio, varicella, influenza.

Travel-specific:

- **Hepatitis A:** all unvaccinated travelers to endemic regions.
- **Hepatitis B:** high-risk (sex exposure, healthcare work, long stays).
- **Typhoid:** South Asia, Africa, Latin America (injectable or oral).
- **Yellow fever:** required for some African/South American countries (certificate may be mandatory).
- **Japanese encephalitis:** rural Asia, long stays, seasonal exposure.
- **Meningococcal:** required for Hajj, sub-Saharan Africa "meningitis belt."
- **Rabies:** for high animal exposure, long rural stays.

Malaria Prevention

Risk assessment: depends on region, duration, rural vs urban.

Chemoprophylaxis (region-specific):

- **Atovaquone-proguanil:** daily, well tolerated.
- **Doxycycline:** daily, also prevents rickettsia/leptospirosis.
- **Mefloquine:** weekly, avoid in psychiatric/seizure disorders.

- **Chloroquine:** only in areas without resistance (rare).

Additional advice:

- Bed nets, insect repellent (DEET/icaridin), long-sleeve clothing.

Other Travel-Related Risks

Traveler's diarrhea:

- Prevention: bottled/boiled water, avoid raw foods, hand hygiene.
- Treatment: oral rehydration, loperamide if mild.
- Consider antibiotics (azithromycin, ciprofloxacin) if severe/prolonged.

Other infections:

- Dengue, chikungunya, Zika: mosquito precautions.
- Schistosomiasis: avoid swimming in freshwater in endemic areas.
- STIs: safe sex counseling.

Environmental risks:

- Altitude sickness: gradual ascent, acetazolamide prophylaxis if needed.
- Jet lag: sleep hygiene, light exposure.

- DVT prevention: compression stockings, ambulation on flights.

When to Refer to Specialists

- Travel medicine clinics for complex itineraries or high-risk patients.
- Infectious disease consultation for immunocompromised travelers or prolonged rural exposure.

Pocket Box – Travel Medicine Quick Reference

- **Assess:** destination, duration, activities, health status.
- **Vaccines:** routine + travel-specific (Hep A/B, typhoid, yellow fever, rabies, meningococcal, JE).
- **Malaria:** chemoprophylaxis (atovaquone-proguanil, doxy, mefloquine, chloroquine).
- **Traveler's diarrhea:** food/water safety, ORS, loperamide ± antibiotics.

Other risks: mosquito protection, STI prevention, altitude/DVT precautions.

Made in United States
North Haven, CT
10 October 2025

80683124R10225